SUPER
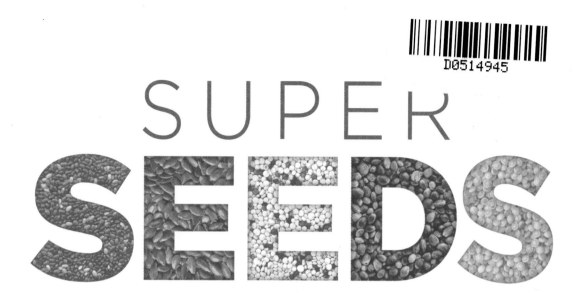
SEEDS

Cooking with Power-Packed
Chia, Quinoa, Flax, Hemp & Amaranth

KIM LUTZ

author of *Welcoming Kitchen*

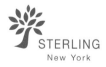

STERLING
New York

For (all) my loving
and supportive parents,
with love and gratitude.

STERLING
New York

An Imprint of Sterling Publishing
387 Park Avenue South
New York, NY 10016

Text © 2014 by Kim Lutz
Photography by Bill Milne
Food styling by Diane Vezza

ISBN 978-1-4549-1278-1

Distributed in Canada by Sterling Publishing
c/o Canadian Manda Group, 165 Dufferin Street
Toronto, Ontario, Canada M6K 3H6
Distributed in the United Kingdom by GMC Distribution Services
Castle Place, 166 High Street, Lewes, East Sussex, England BN7 1XU
Distributed in Australia by Capricorn Link (Australia) Pty. Ltd.
P.O. Box 704, Windsor, NSW 2756, Australia

For information about custom editions, special sales, and premium and corporate purchases, please contact Sterling Special Sales at 800-805-5489 or specialsales@sterlingpublishing.com.

Manufactured in Canada

2 4 6 8 10 9 7 5 3 1

www.sterlingpublishing.com

CONTENTS

We have officially entered the era of super seeds! These days you can find flax just about everywhere, even at your local supermarket. As for chia—it is in everything from juice drinks to gluten-free flours. And don't even get me started on quinoa: Is there any place this Central American super seed hasn't been?

As a superfood author, it's my job to eat, sleep, and live superfoods. So when I noticed an uptick in the popularity of super seeds like hemp and amaranth, whose profile isn't quite as high as chia, quinoa, or flax I paid attention. In *Super Seeds*, Kim Lutz has done a stellar job of introducing us to these important superfoods. Here, you'll learn how each of them can help you feel healthier and re-energized, while enjoying a new way to eat and feel great. The book offers a comprehensive collection of delicious whole food recipes designed to nourish and delight. Kim's breakfast, lunch, dinner, dessert, and snack recipes make it easy to add powerful chia, quinoa, flax, hemp, and amaranth to every meal.

I love Kim's recipe for Quinoa Breakfast Burritos (page 33) and her decadent Chocolate Sunflower Seed–Hemp Butter (page 20) is out of this world! (Try it on pear and apple slices.)

I first came across Kim's work a few years ago on a visit to Sterling, the publisher of this very book. I'd stopped in to see my editor about a book I was working on, *Chia*, also published by Sterling, and which I co-wrote with Dr. Wayne Coates. She excitedly handed me a copy of Kim's earlier book, which Kim had written with Megan Hart, *Welcoming Kitchen: 200 Delicious Allergen & Gluten-free Vegan Recipes*. I took the book home, spent a few nights reading Kim's inviting text, and then tried her recipes for chocolate cake and "throw-together" tomato soup. I loved them!

Indeed, Kim has a reputation for developing healthy recipes that taste great and make sense for the whole family—that's the concept behind a "welcoming kitchen." At Kim's table there is something delicious and safe to eat for everyone. With *Super Seeds*, she turns her attention to chia, quinoa, flax, hemp, and amaranth. This powerful quintet delivers protein, fiber, amino acids, omega-3 fatty acids, and a wide range of vitamins, minerals, and phytonutrients. If you care about getting healthy—and staying healthy—you'll want each of these seeds in your diet. And for those of you (like me) who love to know about the science and research that supports every health claim, you'll be happy to know that there is plenty of evidence to support each of five super seed's individual health benefits.

YOUR HEALTHY HEART

Heart disease is the number one cause of death for both men and women in the United States (and throughout the First World, for that matter) and claims approximately one million lives every year.

Fortunately, lifestyle choices go a long way to help prevent and treat heart disease. One easy thing you can do to keep yourself heart-healthy is to eat foods that are high in omega-3 fatty acids. Research has shown that the omega-3 fatty acid in chia seeds, for example, not only prevents high blood pressure and high cholesterol levels, it also helps lower existing high blood pressure, while reducing total LDL and triglyceride cholesterol in healthy individuals and those diagnosed with cardiovascular disease.

Flax is another rich plant source of omega-3 fatty acids, making it a wonderful superfood for those who are looking to improve cardiovascular health. A review of nine clinical trials suggests that 15–50 grams of flaxseed—either whole or ground—can reduce total LDL cholesterol by 1.6 to 18% in individuals with normal and elevated cholesterol levels.

And not to be left out, quinoa, hemp, and amaranth are no cardiovascular slackers, either. Studies on each of these have found that the oils and fiber in these seeds help lower triglyceride levels while reducing the inflammation in the vessels that contributes to cardiovascular disease. This alone is a good reason to have one or more daily servings of these seeds!

CANCER FIGHTERS

In 2012, 8.2 million people, out of an estimated 14 million people who had cancer, died from the disease. Just as depressing, the World Health Organization predicts that by 2032, new cancer cases will hover around 22 million a year, with 13 million individuals dying of cancer from the disease every year. Choosing cancer-fighting foods—including super seeds—is one way to help lower your risk of becoming a statistic.

The high levels of phytonutrients—such as antioxidants—in chia, quinoa, flax, hemp, and amaranth, help prevent and fight cancer. Antioxidants are chemicals that block the activity of other chemicals known as free radicals, which are highly reactive and have the potential to cause damage to cells that may lead to cancer.

Here's an interesting aside: Here in the United States, there is a lot of talk about using marijuana medically to lessen symptoms of cancer. Hemp, a non-narcotic plant related to marijuana, contains cannabinoids, a family of potent antitumor agents. No fewer than 12 studies by researchers throughout North America and Europe have found that the cannabinoids in hemp help prevent a wide range of cancers and shrink cancerous tumors. What does this mean for you? If cancer prevention is a priority, you might want to consider eating at least one serving of hemp as often as possible. This book has plenty of tempting recipes that will help make healthy dietary adjustments both easy and delicious.

HOT FLASH HELPERS

For many women, hot flashes are an uncomfortable part of life. Once upon a time, many MDs prescribed estrogen replacement therapy to lesson hot flashes. But recently research has found that women who take estrogen replacement therapy are at greater risk of stroke, heart disease, blood clots, and various cancers. Looking for a safer alternative, some women have turned to flaxseed, a plant estrogen. A 2007 Mayo Clinic study backs up the efficiency of flax to relieve hot flashes: 21 women who consumed 40 grams of ground flaxseed a day experienced significant decreases in the frequency and severity of their hot flashes. The women's hot flashes were scored over a period of six weeks. Women who consumed flaxseed showed a 50% decrease in the frequency of hot flashes and a 57% decrease in their "flash score" overall, resulting in major improvements in their quality of life.

BRAIN BOOSTERS

When I first began studying nutrition, one of the things that fascinated me the most about super seeds—such as chia, flax, and hemp—was their ability to help people stabilize mood and focus their attention. Omega-3 fatty acids are known as brain boosters because they are highly concentrated in the brain and appear to be important for memory, as well as mood. Symptoms of omega-3 fatty acid deficiency include fatigue, poor memory, mood swings, and depression.

DIGESTIVE SYSTEM HEALERS

Quinoa, flax, hemp, and amaranth are rich in insoluble fiber, the digestion-helping, bulk-forming, gut-healthy fiber. Unlike soft, gel-like soluble fiber, insoluble fiber does not dissolve or become soft in water, so it passes through the gastrointestinal tract relatively intact, brushing against the wall of your large intestine and scrubbing it clean while it speeds the passage of food and waste through your gut.

DIABETES BUSTERS

According to the International Diabetes Federation, there are approximately 382 million people who are currently living with diabetes. Reliance on simple carbohydrates, such as white bread and crackers, as well as sugary foods, such as soft drinks and candy, has been blamed for the soaring number of diabetes cases around the world.

A large number of studies performed by researchers internationally have found that high-fiber, nutrient-dense foods help to either prevent diabetes and other blood sugar conditions, lessen their severity, or obliterate them altogether. The fiber in chia, quinoa, flax, hemp, and amaranth works to regulate and even lower glucose levels in the blood.

WEIGHT LOSS HELPERS

You know that feeling of satiety you get when you eat certain foods that keep you from snacking a couple of hours after you've eaten a meal? Soluble fiber provides that feeling in a big way, and one of the best sources of soluble fiber I know of is chia. Stir a tablespoon in a glass of water and wait. You'll see the seeds swell, soften, and float like puffy poppy seeds. Incidentally, this is called Chia Fresca. Yes, it's a real drink—and one I prescribe to many of my clients before they go anywhere where they may be tempted to overindulge in nutrient-poor, starchy foods. I think you know what I'm talking about!

The best gateway to enjoy the enormous health benefits of chia, quinoa, flax, hemp, and amaranth is to dive into Kim's delicious recipes and see just how good they make you feel. As you'll see, Kim has provided a wide range of great recipes to entice you. I have no doubt you'll find more than a few new favorites in these pages. You'll also discover how easy it is to whip together the recipes and make super seeds a part of every meal. Happiness and health to you!

Much love,
Stephanie Pedersen, MS, CHHC
Co-writer, with Wayne Coates, PhD,
of *Chia: The Complete Guide to the Ultimate Superfood* and author of *Kale: The Complete Guide to the World's Most Powerful Superfood*
www.StephaniePedersen.com

When I was in college and in my early twenties, I bought into all the hype about the benefits of eating low-fat processed foods and "lite" treats. I must have consumed gallons of chemicals, thinking I was doing the right thing for myself! Little did I know that these foods are actually devoid of any real nutrition. In fact, some manufacturers load up their products—cereals and crackers, for example—with processed sugars and sodium to make them palatable, and use refining processes that actually strip nutrient-rich bran and germ from whole grains, leaving behind only the starchy remainder of the grain.

To improve their image, these manufacturers frequently spray or augment heavily processed foods with a few vitamins and minerals to make the nutritional information panel on their packaging sound appealing. Without fiber, micronutrients, and phytochemicals, however, these products lack the blocks that actually help build healthy bodies.

It was not until the birth of my first child, in 2002, that I became fully aware of the noxious chemicals hidden inside seemingly healthy foods. Within months of my son's birth, it became clear that he had some serious health problems. After much testing and trial and error, we discovered that he has multiple food allergies, a world that we had to learn to navigate quickly, and one that requires a very close reading of food labels, it turns out. When you really look at the long lists of ingredients—many of which are unpronounceable and include scary chemicals—in so many "lite" and "healthy" foods, you can get a powerful shock, especially if you've been eating them on a regular basis, as I had been.

After the food label epiphany, I started really thinking about what I was buying and cooking. To keep my son safe from foods that could harm him, I needed to be careful about what I prepared for him, but I also wanted our whole family to be better nourished. This motivated me to do a lot more home cooking, using a greater variety of fruits and vegetables, whole grains, and legumes. As a result of this experimentation I started feeling better, too—better than I'd ever felt, in fact!

Some of my friends and family who were still eating more standard American foods, however, asked me how my two children could possibly thrive on such a "limited" diet, without meat and dairy products and so few processed and refined convenience foods. When we dined with other people, it seemed to them that we were eating very few things, but in reality our new whole-foods diet had introduced us to an incredible bounty of ingredients that I'd discovered in natural food stores, ethnic markets, and farmers' markets. Rather than shriveling up, my family was flourishing on our new diet.

One of the best and most enduring discoveries I made during my family's journey to healthier eating is a class of seeds that are now being referred to as "super seeds," which includes chia, quinoa, flax, hemp, and amaranth. In my kitchen, these versatile, nutritional powerhouses have found their way into just about every meal and snack of the day, including my family's morning smoothies and even some of our favorite desserts. Super seeds are not only rich in protein and fiber, they also provide a good source of vitamins, minerals, and phytochemicals, including iron, manganese, calcium, and omega-3 and omega-6 fatty acids. I'm confident that once you start experimenting with these tiny, delicious seeds, you'll find them indispensable.

Keep reading and see for yourself!
Kim Lutz

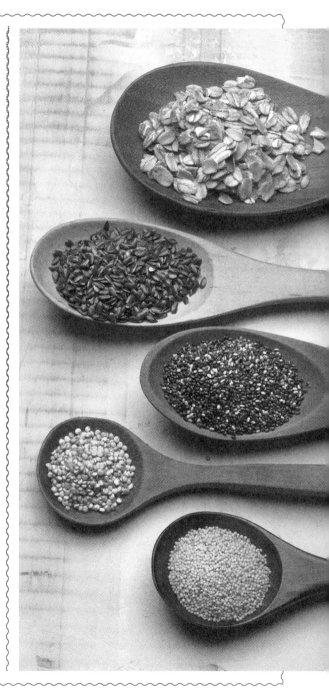

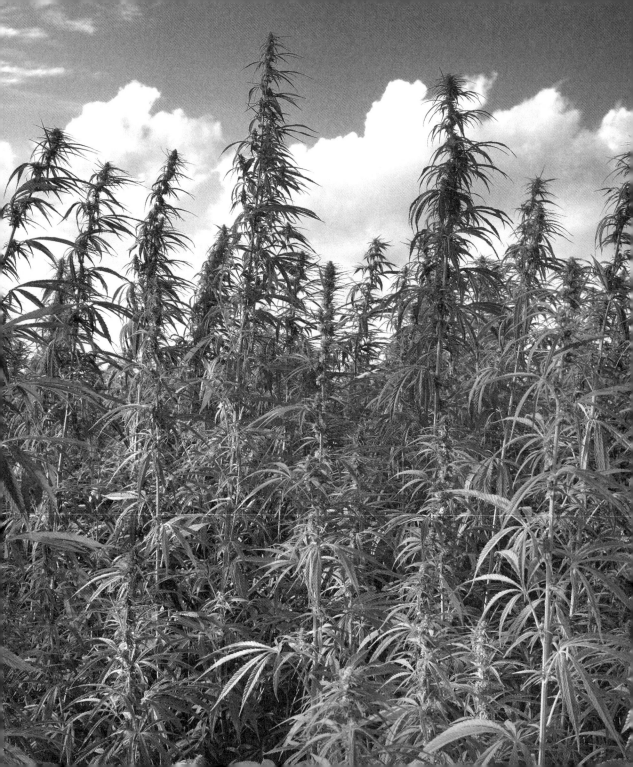

CHAPTER 1

THE POWER OF SUPER SEEDS

Super seeds are itty-bitty powerhouses that aren't just loaded with nutrients, they are popular, versatile players in the kitchen, whether you're enjoying quinoa as a side dish or tossing some flaxseed meal into a batch of breakfast muffins. Super seeds bring something nourishing and delicious to the table every day and at every meal. This chapter explores the astonishing nutrient profiles and health benefits of chia, quinoa, flax, hemp, and amaranth seeds. They all deliver dozens of vitamins and many minerals, plus fiber, antioxidants, fatty acids, amino acids, protein, and much more. Here you'll discover just how powerful these little seeds truly are.

OPPOSITE: **Hemp field**

NUTRITIONAL BENEFITS OF SUPER SEEDS

Our bodies need a range of nutrients to thrive. Luckily, super seeds provide a rich nutritional profile that can translate into vibrant health. Super seeds are wonderful sources of plant protein, which is crucial to cell health throughout the body and helps build strong muscles. Because these powerful little seeds come from plants, all of them are cholesterol-free and low in saturated fat, unlike animal-based protein sources, which have been linked to heart disease and other ailments.

Super seeds make their nutrition available to almost everyone, including people on a restricted diet. And, because they are all naturally gluten free, super seeds are not likely to cause allergic reactions.

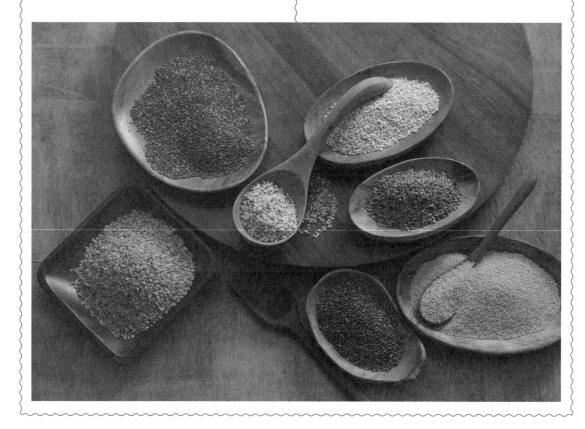

WATER TO THE RESCUE

One of the many benefits of super seeds is their high fiber content. Dietary fiber absorbs liquid in the digestive tract and causes a slower release of the sugars found in food (even natural foods, such as grains, fruits, and seeds). While there are many benefits associated with a higher fiber diet, such as improved digestion, weight control, and more stable blood sugar, eating a higher fiber diet requires plenty of water. If you are following a high-fiber diet, be sure to drink a good amount of water (6 to 8 cups a day is a good goal) so that you are effectively flushing out your system. If you drink too little water, all that fiber can absorb the liquid in your system and cause you to feel bloated and uncomfortable.

WATER SOLUBLE B VITAMINS

Super seeds are rich in B vitamins (including, thiamine, folate, and vitamin B6). B vitamins are water soluble, meaning that our bodies take what they need from them and then excrete the rest in our urine. A great way to ensure that you are getting enough B vitamins for healthy cell function, energy, and overall good health, is to eat dishes containing super seeds, such as the recipes in this book.

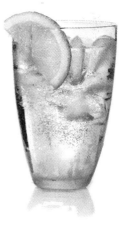

CHIA

The nine essential amino acids in chia make it a high-quality source of protein. One ounce (a little less than 2 tablespoons) of chia delivers a whopping 11 grams of fiber and 4 grams of protein. It's the dietary fiber in chia that helps make it so filling. Many people are turning to chia to achieve or maintain a healthy weight. The fiber in chia keeps you feeling full and allows for a slower breakdown and absorption of food. Chia also can contribute to strong bones with healthy doses of calcium, phosphorus, and manganese.

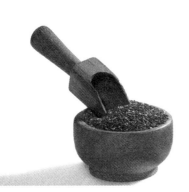

WHAT IS OLD IS NEW

Chia, or *Salvia hispanica*, is a member of the mint family. Historically, it was grown and consumed in Mexico, where it fueled the Aztec Empire for centuries. The powerful nutrition provided by the tiny seed (protein, minerals, and fiber) supplied long-distance runners and warriors with a superb, long-lasting source of fuel, and today it remains a reliable source of energy.

* * *

THE BEAUTY OF GOO— USING SOAKED CHIA

Although chia seeds are tiny they can get stuck in your teeth, and because they absorb nine times their weight in water, they can get gooey pretty quickly. This can feel very weird! This absorptive quality is a benefit to cooking, though, because chia seeds mixed with water become gelatinous. Be sure to give chia seeds a good soak if you are using them to replace eggs. Soak them for at least 10 minutes in water, and make sure to stir the mixture so that there are no dry seeds. You can also grind chia seeds in a nut and seed grinder or a clean coffee grinder before using them. If you use chia seeds in a smoothie, be sure to blend them in well.

QUINOA

There's a reason this South American seed is at the top of so many superfood lists. One cup of cooked quinoa has 8 grams of complete protein and 5 grams of dietary fiber. Amino acids are the building blocks of protein. Essential amino acids are the amino acids that must come from our food, since our bodies are unable to produce them. Quinoa is rich in several of these essential amino acids, making it an excellent source of plant-based protein. Since quinoa is cholesterol-free and also full of fiber, it is a healthy alternative to animal-based sources of protein, including meat and cows' milk. In addition, quinoa contains more than 10 percent of the dietary recommended daily allowance for a wide range of vitamins that includes thiamin, riboflavin, vitamin B6, and folate, and it is packed with minerals such as, iron, magnesium, phosphorus, zinc, copper, and manganese

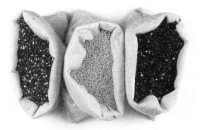

A SUPER START FOR BABY

Amaranth and quinoa porridge are wonderful first solids for babies because they are not likely to cause an allergic reaction, they cook up smooth, and are easy to sweeten naturally. Try mixing in mashed banana or sweet potato. You may end up eating more of this porridge than your baby!

* * *

THE SOFT SIDE OF QUINOA FLOUR

Quinoa flour can have a grassy taste and aroma. A little bit of it mixed into a flour blend can complement a dish, depending on the other flavors. If you're not crazy about the "grassiness" of the flavor, however, you can toast quinoa flour by spreading it on a rimmed baking sheet and heating it in a 225°F oven for 2 to 3 hours. (You don't need to stir it while it's heating.) You'll know it's done when the grassy smell is gone.

FLAX

Ground flaxseed is an excellent source of fiber (each tablespoon contains about 8 grams) as well as a good source of magnesium, phosphorus, copper, thiamin, and manganese. Also, since flax can be used to take the place of eggs, it is particularly helpful to folks who need to watch their intake of dietary cholesterol. In fact, all five super seeds are cholesterol-free. Whole flaxseed is encased in a very tough exterior, however, making it indigestible unless it is ground. Because it can pass through the digestive system intact, however, some people use whole flaxseed as a laxative. In addition, flax—and hemp seed, as well—is a very good source of plant-based omega-3 fatty acids, which play a role in protecting against inflammation and high blood pressure.

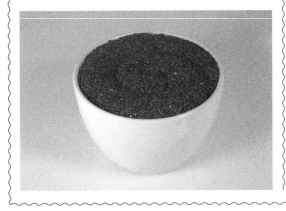

FLAXSEED VS. FLAXSEED MEAL

The nutrients in flaxseed aren't accessible in their whole form, but if you grind the seed into meal, you'll get all the benefits—protein, fiber, and minerals. If you don't want to bother with grinding your own meal, no worries: You can easily purchase ground or milled flax at your local health food store and many mainstream grocery stores. Once you buy it, make sure it is tightly sealed and keep it in the freezer to keep it from turning rancid.

* * *

FLAXSEED AND YOUR FURRY FRIEND

Flax really is good for the whole family, including your favorite canine. Add a little flaxseed meal or flaxseed oil to dog food to help give your pooch a shiny coat and a healthy digestive system. Before you add flaxseed to your pet's diet, however, be sure to ask your veterinarian if it is a good supplement for your pet.

HEMP

Hemp seed is loaded with protein. Just one ounce (3 tablespoons) of shelled hemp seeds contains more than 10 grams of protein. You can eat either whole hemp seed or shelled hemp seed. I prefer shelled, or hulled, hemp seeds (also called hemp hearts) because they are easier to eat. (Although the hull also contains nutrients, it is fibrous, crunchy, and a bit hard to chew.) Hemp seeds taste nutty and have a nutty texture, and since they are seeds, they are a great alternative to nuts for people who are nut allergic. Not only are hemp seeds loaded with protein (2 tablespoons have 10 grams of protein) they are also a good source of other important nutrients including iron, magnesium, and zinc, all of which are crucial minerals for good health.

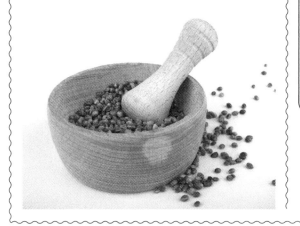

CAN HEMP SEEDS GET YOU HIGH?

Although hemp seeds are related to marijuana, they are not considered a drug because hemp seeds, and foods made from hemp, contain at most miniscule amounts of THC, the psychoactive component of marijuana. Healthy eating might make you feel good, but it's not the same "high" as from marijuana!

* * *

LOVELY IN HEMP

There are many reasons to look to hemp as a fabric of choice when choosing your clothing. Where conventional cotton uses huge amounts of pesticides to grow, hemp grows well in almost any climate without the need for extra pesticides and herbicides. Its roots can grow several feet deep, which helps promote healthy soil by preventing run-off. Not only is hemp fiber good for the environment, it makes for a very durable cloth, so your clothes can last longer, too!

AMARANTH

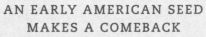

This seed truly is the king of all seeds when it comes to protein. One cup of cooked amaranth contains more than 9 grams of protein. Unlike a lot of other plant-based proteins, amaranth contains all the amino acids (the building blocks of protein) that we need, making it a complete protein. Amaranth is also a good source of fiber (5.2 grams per cup), unlike animal proteins. When you consider the vitamins and minerals that are packed into this grainlike seed, you can't help but be wowed. One cup of cooked amaranth contains more than 10 percent of the RDA (recommended daily allowance) of vitamin B6, folate, calcium, iron, zinc, copper, and selenium; and it is a fantastic source of magnesium, phosphorus, and manganese. And amaranth is gluten-free.

AN EARLY AMERICAN SEED MAKES A COMEBACK

Amaranth was a thriving crop and a staple of the Aztec diet hundreds of years ago, but when the Spaniards brought Catholicism to Mexico, it was banned because Aztec people used it (along with human blood) in the sacrifices they made to their gods. Because of amaranth's impressive nutritional profile—it's a rich source of high-quality protein, amino acids, iron, potassium, calcium, and manganese—efforts by the nonprofit group Mexico Tierra de Amaranto are now under way to bring this super seed back into gardens and kitchens, and onto dinner plates once again. The group is also focused on improving working conditions for rural Mexican farmers through amaranth cultivation.

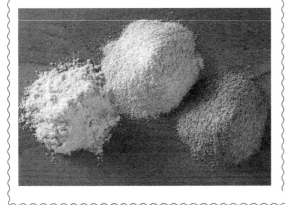

VITAMINS, MINERALS AND OTHER IMPORTANT CHEMICAL ELEMENTS IN SUPER SEEDS

VITAMIN B6   B6 is necessary for more than 100 enzyme reactions and is involved in metabolism, brain development, and immune function.

FOLATE   A form of vitamin B, Folate is necessary for cell division and DNA synthesis.

CALCIUM   Calcium contributes to strong bones, helps muscles move, sends messages through the nerves, and helps blood circulation.

ZINC   Zinc helps the immune system fight off invading bacteria and viruses; it also helps heal wounds.

COPPER   Copper helps form strong and flexible connective tissue. It also plays a critical role in cellular energy production.

SELENIUM   Selenium is important for reproduction (a deficit may contribute to male infertility), thyroid function, and protecting the body from infection.

MAGNESIUM   Magnesium contributes to bone formation.

PHOSPHORUS   Phosphorus is important for bone health, DNA and RNA formation, and for oxygen delivery to body tissues.

MANGANESE   Manganese is a component of many essential enzymes that work with bone development, metabolism, and wound healing.

THIAMINE   Also known as vitamin B_1, thiamine helps our bodies convert carbohydrates into fuel. It also contributes to a strong immune system.

IRON   Iron is essential for a healthy body. It helps metabolize protein and contributes to healthy blood.

WHOLE FOODS SAVE THE DAY

Being selective about the foods you eat—avoiding processed foods, for example—is the most direct way to stay healthy. The removal of refined and unhealthy products from your diet will help ensure that your body has all the nutrients it needs to thrive. Here, again, super seeds play a superhero role.

The traditional Standard American Diet (SAD—and that's not only an acronym!) is replete with processed foods in which the nutrients have been stripped away. They might taste good and satisfy our hunger over the short term, but they don't provide what our bodies need to thrive over the long run. This is where super seeds step in to provide whole-food alternatives to overprocessed and nutritionally stripped-down foods. Quinoa, for example, cooks quickly and easily and makes an ideal substitute for white rice. In 15 minutes you can have a fluffy base for a stir-fry or main-dish salad. If you're looking for a healthy alternative to instant (and sugar-filled) hot cereals, make a pot of amaranth, keep it in the refrigerator in a sealed container, and warm it up with fruit and nondairy milk.

Are you looking for cholesterol-free egg substitutes for recipes? Look no further than chia or ground flaxseed! Chia seeds and flaxseed form a gel when they're mixed with water, making them an excellent substitute for eggs in both savory and sweet dishes—without the cholesterol and saturated fat! Of course, with the addition of chia or ground flaxseed—to anything you eat—you are also getting beneficial fiber.

Adding whole-food ingredients such as quinoa or amaranth flour to gluten-free flour blends will increase the nutrition of your baked goods. Many commercial all-purpose gluten-free flour blends rely on white rice flour and tapioca starch. Although these grains may provide an appealing texture, they are fairly devoid of nutrients. To address the nutritional deficit, mix in some protein-, fiber- and mineral-rich super seed flour. It's easy to substitute ¼ cup of quinoa or amaranth flour for ¼ cup of all-purpose gluten-free flour mix for each cup of flour you need. You don't want to trade out more than ¼ cup per cup, though, because the flavors of these flours can be a little overpowering.

Another whole food—hemp seeds—can literally be a lifesaver for folks who have nut allergies. Just as their name implies, hemp seeds are seeds and not nuts. Therefore, they are safe to serve, in every form and preparation, to people who are allergic to nuts and peanuts. The fat and protein profile in hemp seeds is similar to nuts. They're creamy when they're blended, they bake up nice and crunchy, and even add a dash of nutty flavor. Hemp seeds can also be combined with sunflower seeds or shelled pumpkin seeds (pepitas) for another variation on nut-free crunch. In addition, hemp seeds are a good substitution for nuts in nondairy milk and nut-butter recipes.

All-purpose flour, white rice, vegetable oil, and margarine dominate the Standard American Diet. Using super seeds to make small changes can transform favorite dishes into health-promoting meals, however. The recipes in this book show you how you can use whole-grain flours, seed flours, cooked amaranth and quinoa, chia gel, and flaxseed meal to create this nutrition revolution. Instead of relying on ingredients with stripped-away nutrition, you can use these easy-to-use seeds to

WHAT'S SO GOOD ABOUT FIBER?

Chia, quinoa, flax, hemp, and amaranth are all good sources of fiber. Why is fiber so necessary? For one, we need fiber in our diet because it plays an important role in our digestive health. Fiber adds bulk to food, which slows down the rate at which food is absorbed. This process makes it easier for waste to pass through the bowels and can even help play a role in regulating blood sugar (and lowering your risk of diabetes). Also, fiber helps you feel full after eating, which makes it less likely that you'll overeat. Need another reason? Recent studies have shown that high-fiber diets can help lower cholesterol and therefore your risk of heart disease.

* * *

HOW MUCH PROTEIN DO I REALLY NEED?

Protein-rich super seeds can play an important role in a well-rounded diet. Protein is an essential component of cell health. The amount of protein you need often depends on a combination of factors, such as your age and lifestyle; whether you exercise frequently; or if you are trying to lose weight, etc. A good rule of thumb? About 15 to 20 percent of your calories should come from protein.

pump up the vitamins, minerals, protein, and fiber in every meal.

Any vegetarian can tell you that he or she is frequently asked, "Where do you get your protein?" Super seeds provides an answer. For example, just adding amaranth to polenta turns a comforting dish into a complete meal. Here's why: Although polenta—cornmeal that is boiled into a porridge and then prepared in various ways—is tasty all on its own, the protein in cornmeal does not contain a full range of amino acids. If you add amaranth to cornmeal, however, you will get all the benefits of a complete protein. Another way to give baked goods a nutrient boost is to swap out a percentage of ordinary cooking oil with fiber-, protein-, and mineral-rich flax seed meal. Cooking oil doesn't contain any protein or fiber, but if you replace some of the oil with flaxseed meal, you'll get a more nutrient-dense dish. Your cookies or muffins will not only be healthier for you, they'll have a richer, nuttier flavor as well.

At every meal, super seeds keep you energized, and also make a great mid-afternoon snack whenever you need a little extra push to get you through the day. If you love smoothies, try adding hemp, chia, or flaxseed to the mix for a super creamy drink that also gives you a healthy dash of fiber.

As a natural thickener, chia is the perfect, whole-food choice for making delicious jellies, syrups, and puddings without using nutritionally empty starches or animal-derived gelatin. And, since chia can thicken even cold liquids, it is ideal for raw food preparations. Instead of cranking up your stove and heating up the house on a hot day, use chia to thicken sauces and gravies. You can also use flaxseed to add both thickness and a nutritional boost to savory liquids.

The recipes in this book use whole grains and unrefined sweeteners, along with a colorful array of fruits and vegetables, and of course super seeds. With this combination of nourishing, delicious ingredients, every meal can be super!

Starting with basic preparations and moving through breakfasts, soups and salads, entrees, baked goods, and desserts, this cookbook can help you to transform your meals—and your well-being.

HELP FOR KIDS WITH CELIAC DISEASE

Lara Field, MS, RD, CSP, LDN, a pediatric dietitian who works closely with children diagnosed with celiac disease, has pointed out that "amaranth is a wonderful addition to a gluten-free diet, because it is a rich source of many vitamins and minerals, including vitamin B6, folate, iron, magnesium, phosphorus, and manganese," nutrients that are typically consumed in lower quantities with a gluten-free diet. Amaranth, however, is "a fantastic replacement," she adds, for missing B vitamins and iron.

* * *

SUPER SEEDS AND THEIR ROLE IN AMERICAN HISTORY

The Constitution and the Bill of Rights were written on parchment (an animal skin that has been prepared for printing or writing). However, since most paper at the time of the writing of these documents (1787) was made of hemp or flax, it is probable that early drafts of these important documents were written on the fiber of super-seed plants!

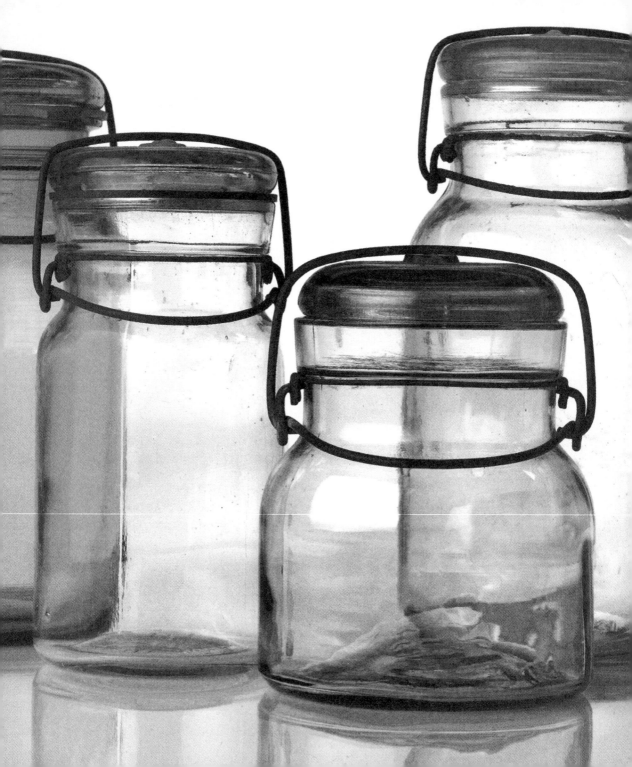

CHAPTER 2

BASIC SUPER SEED RECIPES AND PREPARATIONS

Many ingredient lists in this book include more than one seed in order to give the recipes an extra nutritional boost. This chapter covers everything you need to know about basic super seed recipes and the simple tools you'll need to use super seeds in various forms, whether it is flour, a seed butter, or nondairy milk. You'll also discover what to keep on hand to serve, store, and reuse basic super seed preparations.

OPPOSITE: **Antique glass storage jars**

EASY INTRODUCTIONS

Getting started with chia, flax, hemp, quinoa, and amaranth is practically effortless. You can begin by sprinkling flaxseed meal or shelled hemp seeds onto yogurt or fruit, or tossing some quinoa or amaranth into soup as it's cooking to add texture, protein, fiber, vitamins, and minerals—all of which are abundant in these tiny, nutritional powerhouses. You'll enjoy their nutty flavor and also be surprised by how quickly you'll feel the health benefits of including super seeds in your diet.

One of the easiest and tastiest ways to make super seeds a welcome addition to the family dinner table is to gradually replace rice with quinoa or amaranth. As you'll discover, super seeds are incredibly versatile and easy to work into just about every meal, including snacks and desserts. They are a bit like a blank canvas that you can color with an infinite variety of flavors. In this book, you'll find basic recipes for chia, quinoa, flax, hemp and amaranth. You'll also learn how to make a nut-butter alternative, a nondairy milk, and an egg substitute.

USEFUL KITCHEN SUPPLIES

Having some basic kitchen utensils on hand can help you make the most of cooking with super seeds. Here are some items I always have in my kitchen:

- Blender
- Food processor
- Nut and seed grinder or coffee grinder
- Strainer or fine-mesh colander (to rinse quinoa)
- Parchment paper (for easy baking cleanup)
- Sheet pans
- Muffin tins and cake pans
- Lidded saucepan (for cooking quinoa and amaranth)
- Large baking dish/lasagna pan (9 × 13)
- Clean jars with lids (to store bulk seeds, hemp milk, seed butters, etc.)
- Freezer-safe containers to store leftovers and keep flaxseed fresh (in the freezer for up to 6 months)

GRINDING YOUR OWN SEED FLOURS

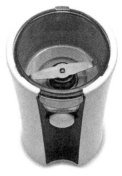

Although you can purchase quinoa and amaranth flours that are already perfectly milled and ready to use, it's easy to use a clean coffee or nut grinder to transform quinoa or amaranth into a fine flour. More often than not, you'll see this method used to grind whole flaxseed into flaxseed meal. And if you want to use chia without the tapioca-like texture of soaked chia, you can grind the seeds into flour as well—a process that will yield a smoother gel when the flour is combined with water or other liquids. However, I prefer to use chia as an egg substitute (see Chapter 3); to make puddings, smoothies, and syrups; or almost anything that can be enhanced by chia seeds' gel-like properties. Hemp seeds are tiny, making them ideal to use whole or ground into a delicious butter (see Sunflower Hemp Seed Butter later in this chapter) or soak them in water to make a milk (see Hemp Milk later in this chapter).

* * *

HOW TO USE SUPER SEED FLOUR
WITH ALL-PURPOSE FLOUR

For every cup of all-purpose flour, substitute ¼ cup of seed flour. Keep in mind that using too much of a seed flour can significantly alter the texture and flavor of the finished product. Quinoa, and to a lesser extent amaranth flour, can have a grassy flavor, which you can improve by toasting the flour in a 225°F oven for 2 to 3 hours. It's important to keep in mind that seed flours are gluten-free. Gluten is the component of wheat flour that binds molecules together. So if you are baking with quinoa or amaranth flour, you will need to combine it with a gluten-containing flour or oat flour, which has similar properties to wheat flour, but can be gluten-free. Or you can use a gluten-free binder such as xanthan gum or guar gum. Otherwise, your baked goods will not hold together.

BASIC QUINOA

MAKES 2 CUPS

Quinoa seeds have a soapy, bitter-tasting coating (to keep birds from eating them), but a thorough rinse makes it is easy to remove the strong taste. Most quinoa sold in the United States is pre-rinsed, but if you have any doubts, just put it in a strainer and rinse the quinoa until the water runs clear.

> *2 cups water or broth*
> *Pinch of salt (optional)*
> *1 cup quinoa (rinsed, if necessary)*

1. Combine water or broth, optional salt, and quinoa in a small saucepan over medium-high heat and bring to a boil.
2. Cover, reduce heat, and simmer for 15 minutes or until the liquid is absorbed and the outer coat spirals off the quinoa. (The mixture will look like a lot of little commas.)
3. Fluff with a fork before serving.

BASIC AMARANTH

MAKES 3 CUPS

Amaranth is a smaller seed than quinoa, and it has a smoother texture when it's cooked.

> *3 cups water or broth*
> *Pinch of salt (optional)*
> *1 cup amaranth*

1. Combine water or broth, optional salt, and amaranth in a small saucepan over medium-high heat and bring to a boil.
2. Cover, reduce heat, and simmer for 25 to 30 minutes, or until liquid is absorbed.
3. Fluff with a fork before serving.

QUINOA GETS ITS 15 MINUTES OF FAME

The United Nations declared 2013 the International Year of Quinoa. (It is only the second food to earn a UN international observance. The first food was rice in 2004.) According to United Nations Food and Agriculture Organization Director-General José Graziano da Silva, quinoa can play an important role in eradicating hunger, malnutrition, and poverty. The International Year of Quinoa highlighted quinoa's strong nutritional profile and its ability to grow in arid conditions and varied temperatures, such as in Africa.

POPPED AMARANTH

YIELDS ABOUT ¼ CUP

Popping increases the volume by about 3 times, and popped amaranth will look like tiny kernels of popcorn. A great way to raise the nutritional profile of your breakfast is to mix ¼ cup popped amaranth with ¾ cup crisp brown-rice cereal and serve it with nondairy milk (a combination of hemp milk and almond milk, for example)—a tasty way to add more super seed goodness to your breakfast bowl. Add some sliced strawberries, and you have a tasty, filling, and nutritious to start to the day. I like to make several batches of popped amaranth one at a time, and then store it in a sealed jar for use over the next couple of days as a topping to sprinkle over yogurt or a salad or to eat straight from the jar. Delicious.

5 teaspoons amaranth seeds

1. Heat a large saucepan over medium-high heat.

2. When a drop of water immediately balls up on the dry pan surface, add amaranth seeds and distribute them evenly over the bottom of the pan in a single layer. Cover and turn off heat. Most of the amaranth will pop, though the unpopped seeds can still be eaten and will have a nice toasty flavor and crunch.

3. Pour the popped amaranth into a bowl and serve with a drizzle of olive oil and a sprinkle of salt.

AMARANTH'S RISING PROFILE

Over the next few years, you can expect amaranth to become as popular as quinoa—they're both very old, high-protein plants with roots in South America; and like quinoa, amaranth is a nutrition force to be reckoned with. Both are rich in quality protein, minerals, and fiber, and of course they're gluten-free. Among its many selling points, in addition to amaranth's super seed status, is its versatility in the kitchen—it is an easy and delicious ingredient to add to just about anything, from salads and stews to soups and desserts. Behind the push to bring amaranth into the spotlight is the Amaranth Institute, a nonprofit organization that acts to collect and disseminate information about amaranth.

SUNFLOWER HEMP SEED BUTTER

MAKES 1 CUP

Although you can enjoy hemp seed butter on its own, I prefer mixing it with sunflower seeds to make a creamier, earthier peanut butter alternative. You can also substitute almonds, cashews, or peanuts for the sunflower seeds in this recipe. For an alternative all-seed version of this delicious butter, replace the sunflower seeds with shelled pumpkin seeds (pepitas).

1 cup raw sunflower seeds
1 cup shelled hemp seeds
   Optional: Pinch of salt, to taste
   Optional: Drizzle of neutral oil, such as canola, grapeseed, or sunflower, to taste
   Optional: Dash of natural sweetener, such as maple syrup, to taste

1. Preheat oven to 350°F.
2. Spread seeds in a thin layer on a rimmed baking sheet.
3. Bake 5 to 10 minutes, until seeds are fragrant and slightly soft but not burned.
4. When the seeds have cooled, grind them into a paste in a food processor or blender, scraping down the sides as necessary, 5 to 10 minutes, or until a smooth, buttery consistency is achieved.
5. Scoop butter into a sealed container. Keep refrigerated for up to one week.

CHOCOLATE SUNFLOWER SEED–HEMP BUTTER

MAKES APPROXIMATELY ¼ CUP

You can drizzle a little water into this decadent-tasting spread if you would like a thinner consistency. Just be sure to blend it well. You can store this seed butter in a covered container in the refrigerator for up to one week.

1 pitted Medjool date
½ cup Sunflower Seed–Hemp Butter (see recipe at left)
1 tablespoon cocoa powder
½ teaspoon vanilla
   pinch of salt

1. Blend all ingredients in a food processor or blender until smooth.

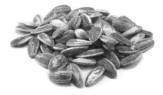

HEMP PESTO

MAKES 1 CUP

Hemp's nutty texture and delicate flavor make it an ideal addition to various pestos, including this variation on classic basil pesto.

½ cup hemp seeds
4 cups basil leaves
½ cup olive oil
4 shallot cloves, minced
1 teaspoon salt
Freshly ground black pepper

1. In a dry skillet over medium heat, toast hemp seeds for 1 to 2 minutes, until seeds are fragrant.
2. Puree all ingredients in a food processor or blender.
3. Store in a sealed container in the refrigerator for up to 3 days.

HEMP MILK

MAKES APPROXIMATELY 6 CUPS

It seems as if the nondairy milk section of the grocery store expands every week. Although it's wonderful to have the option to buy so many products, there is nothing easier than making your own hemp milk. You can use this in any recipe that calls for nondairy milk. If you want to enjoy it as a beverage, try adding a little salt, sweetener and/or vanilla. By making your own nondairy milk you have complete control over the ingredients. Instead of a bunch of stuff you don't want (preservatives, additives, gums, etc.) you'll have a tasty beverage bursting with protein, iron, and magnesium. You can also change the taste of your hemp milk by blending it with another nondairy milk, such as almond or coconut milk.

1 cup hemp seeds
5 to 6 cups water (depending on how creamy you want the milk to be)

1. Blend all ingredients together.
2. Store extra milk in a sealed container in the refrigerator for up to 3 days. Shake before using.

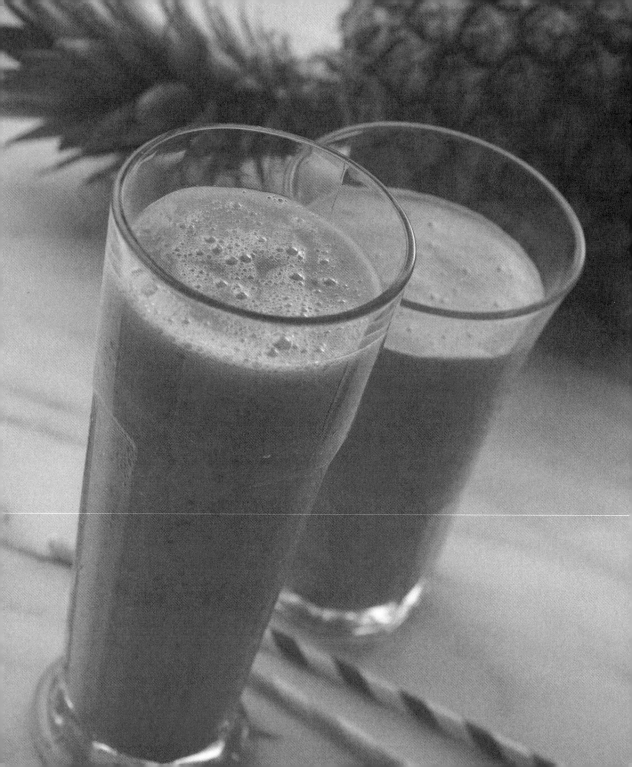

CHAPTER 3

BREAKFASTS

Remember your mom saying that breakfast is the most important meal of the day? Whether one meal is really that much more important than any other is open for debate, but there is no question that adding super seeds to the first meal of the day is a sure way to get off to a good start. The fiber in super seeds will make you feel full so that you don't need to snack before lunch, while the protein and nutrients in these little powerhouses will fuel your breakfast with all the energy you need to accomplish whatever you set out to do.

OPPOSITE: **Carrot Sweet Potato Yogurt Smoothie, page 27, foreground; Vibrant Yogurt Smoothie, page 31, background**

BREAKFAST PANCAKES

MAKES APPROXIMATELY 16 PANCAKES

Pancakes are a favorite weekend breakfast for my family. You can dress them up with fresh fruit (blueberries or diced strawberries are nice) or even add chocolate chips to the batter! If you make a big batch of these pancakes on Sunday, you can wrap any leftovers in foil, pop them in the fridge, and toast them for a special (yet quick) Monday morning treat.

- 2 *tablespoons chia seeds*
- 6 *tablespoons water*
- ½ *cup amaranth flour*
- 2 *cups white whole-wheat flour*
- ¼ *cup coconut palm sugar or evaporated cane juice*
- 2 *teaspoons baking powder*
- 2 *teaspoons baking soda*
- ¼ *teaspoon salt*
- 2½ *cups Hemp Milk (page 21) or other nondairy milk*
- 1 *teaspoon vanilla extract*
- 2 *teaspoons neutral-tasting oil (canola, grapeseed, or sunflower)*

1. In a large bowl, combine chia seeds and water. Set aside.

2. In a medium bowl, combine flours, sugar, baking powder, baking soda, and salt with a whisk.

3. Add nondairy milk, vanilla, and oil to chia mixture. Combine well.

4. Slowly mix dry ingredients into wet mixture. Stir until just combined.

5. Lightly oil a skillet or griddle. Heat over medium heat until a drop of water dances across the surface.

6. Pour approximately ¼ cup of the batter onto the skillet or griddle. Cook until bubbles form in the middle of the pancake.

7. Flip the pancake and cook until both sides are golden brown.

8. Repeat with remaining batter. Don't overcrowd the pan; make sure there is space around pancakes while they cook.

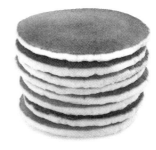

EVAPORATED CANE JUICE:
A SWEETENER THAT'S A LITTLE LESS REFINED

Evaporated cane juice is a sugar made from sugar cane that has been crushed and strained. The liquid is then boiled to evaporate the water, leaving sugar crystals behind. These crystals are less refined than table sugar, and retain small amounts of vitamins and minerals that were present in the sugar cane and are lost in table sugar. The more minimal processing leaves the sugar with an amber cast not present in the more refined table sugar. Organic evaporated cane juice is produced from sugar cane that is grown in accordance with the USDA Organic guidelines. Although slightly more nutrient-rich than table sugar, you should still use sparingly and look to whole foods, like fruits, vegetables, and seeds for your vitamins and minerals, and use sugars of any kind for a sweet treat.

COCONUT PALM SUGAR VS. TABLE SUGAR

Coconut palm sugar is the dehydrated nectar of the flower from the coconut palm tree. Although there is some controversy about whether it is any "better" for you than other sweeteners, the trip from tree to table doesn't involve a lot of steps. In fact, it is one of the least refined sweeteners available. There is also some evidence that coconut palm sugar might be lower on the glycemic index than other sweeteners, but the jury is still out on this point. Coconut palm sugar has more nutrients than cane sugar, but unless you are consuming a lot of sweetener, it probably won't make that much of a difference in your nutritional intake. There are other reasons to consider it, however. Using traditional harvesting methods, the coconut palm tree can produce sugar for up to 20 years, making it a relatively sustainable sweetener. If you're curious about other natural, granulated sweeteners, give date or maple sugar a try.

BLUEBERRY CHIA SYRUP

MAKES 1 CUP

This syrup can be made with any of your favorite fruits. Adding chia to the mix thickens it to a stick-to-the-pancake consistency. Although you don't need to grind chia seeds for this recipe, the syrup will be smoother if you do. (See page 17 for information on grinding chia.)

1½ cups blueberries
½ cup water
2 teaspoons chia seeds
  Optional: Natural sweetener, to taste

1. In a small saucepan, combine blueberries and water. Bring to a boil.

2. Reduce heat. Simmer blueberries until they are soft enough to mash easily with a fork or potato masher.

3. Stir in sweetener, if using, until it dissolves.

4. Turn off heat. Stir in chia seeds. Let mixture rest for at least 10 minutes.

5. Stir again before serving.

IS WHITE WHOLE WHEAT HAVING AN IDENTITY CRISIS?

The question whether white whole wheat is a whole grain or a white (refined) one can finally be put to rest. It is a whole grain. Traditional whole wheat, with its tan color and hearty flavor, comes from red wheat. White whole wheat is lighter in texture and flavor and comes from a white wheat plant. When it is ground from the whole grain, the nutrients in the outer bran are kept intact as opposed to being stripped away, which occurs when the grain is processed for white all-purpose flour.

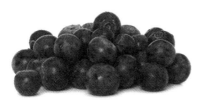

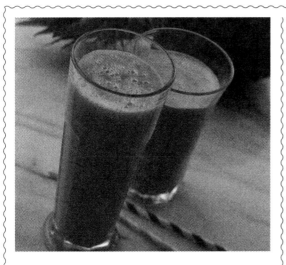

CARROT SWEET POTATO YOGURT SMOOTHIE

MAKES ABOUT 8 CUPS

This smoothie has a lovely peachy golden color. If your blender is not particularly powerful, you can grate the carrots first in a food processor, then add them to the blender. The amounts in the ingredient list are approximate, since carrots and sweet potatoes vary in size. Depending on how thick you want your smoothie to be, you may also want to adjust the amount of nondairy milk and apple juice.

1 sweet potato, peeled and baked

3 carrots, cut into chunks

¾ cup frozen pineapple chunks

¾ cup frozen mango chunks

2 tablespoons chia seeds

1 large dollop (about ¾ cup) nondairy vanilla yogurt

¾ cup Hemp Milk (page 21) or other nondairy milk

¾ cup apple juice

1. Put all ingredients into a blender and process until all ingredients are well blended.

NATURALLY SWEET SMOOTHIES

Of course you could add sugar to your smoothies to sweeten them up a bit, but depending on the season and the types of fruit that are available, your smoothie might not need any extra sweetness at all! If you do want a little extra blast of sweetness, however, try adding some of these naturally sweet ingredients—and toss the sugar!

- dates
- applesauce
- fruit
- stevia
- maple syrup

BLUEBERRY OATMEAL

MAKES 2 SERVINGS

It's so easy to customize your oatmeal with wholesome ingredients, you might never make instant oatmeal again!

- ¼ *cup shelled hemp seeds*
- ½ *cup rolled oats (also called old-fashioned oats, gluten-free if necessary)*
- ½ *cup blueberries*
  Drizzle of maple syrup
  Hemp milk or other nondairy milk, to taste

1. Toast hemp seeds in a dry skillet over medium heat for a minute or two, until the seeds are golden brown.
2. In a medium saucepan, bring oats and 1 cup water to a boil.
3. Reduce heat and simmer 3 to 5 minutes, or until oatmeal is desired consistency.
4. To serve, garnish cooked oatmeal with toasted hemp seeds and blueberries.
5. Drizzle a little maple syrup over the top and add a splash of nondairy milk.

> ### DID YOU KNOW...
> Blueberries are not only in the same botanical family as cranberries and lingonberries—Ericaceae (Heath family)—they are also related to azalea, rhododendron, heather, and heath (hence the family name).

MANGO PINEAPPLE SMOOTHIE

MAKES 4 SERVINGS

Chia adds creaminess and keeps the ingredients from separating in this delicious, tropical-fruit-flavored smoothie. If you don't drink all of it at once, you can store the rest in a sealed jar in the refrigerator for a day. Just give the smoothie a quick shake before you drink it. It will be a little thinner the next day, but you can always blend it with a little ice to bring it back to the milkshake consistency of the first day.

- 1 *cup frozen pineapple chunks*
- 1 *cup frozen mango chunks*
- 2 *carrots, peeled and grated*
- 2 *teaspoons chia seeds*
- ½ *to 1 cup apple juice*
- 1 *to 2 cups Hemp Milk (page 21) or other nondairy milk, to taste, depending on desired consistency*

1. Put all ingredients into a blender and process until well blended.

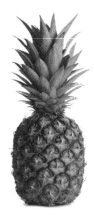

PUMPKIN PANCAKES

MAKES 12 PANCAKES

Whole-grain oat flour makes these pancakes sweet and pillowy—they are just as delicious with gluten-free oat flour.

- ½ cup pumpkin puree (or canned pumpkin)
- 2 tablespoons maple syrup
- 1 cup Hemp Milk (page 21) or other nondairy milk
- 1 tablespoon chia seeds
- 1½ cups (gluten-free) oat flour
- ½ cup flaxseed meal
- 2 teaspoons baking powder
- 2 teaspoons baking soda
- ¼ teaspoon salt
- ¼ teaspoon nutmeg
- 1 teaspoon cinnamon
- 2 teaspoons neutral-tasting oil (canola, grapeseed, or sunflower)

1. In a large bowl, combine pumpkin puree, maple syrup, nondairy milk, and chia. Set aside for 10 minutes.

2. In a medium bowl, use a whisk to combine oat flour, flaxseed meal, baking powder, baking soda, salt, nutmeg, and cinnamon.

3. Add dry ingredients to the wet mixture. Stir to combine.

4. Lightly brush a skillet or griddle with oil. Heat skillet or griddle over medium heat until a drop of water dances on the surface.

5. Scoop batter onto the surface of skillet. Cook until bubbles form in the middle of the pancake and the edges are set.

6. Flip and cook until set on the other side.

7. Repeat steps with remaining batter.

DO OATS CONTAIN GLUTEN?

Gluten, the protein found in wheat, barley, rye, and spelt, binds molecules together and creates a nice crumb. For people who cannot eat gluten, either due to celiac disease or gluten intolerance, all gluten-containing grains must be avoided. Oats contain a protein (avenin) that acts like gluten but is not gluten. For many people who need to avoid gluten, oats are safe to eat *if they are certified gluten-free.* If you avoid gluten, it is important to check with your doctor before adding oats to your diet, because the protein in oats can also be problematic for some people. In addition, almost all oats and oat products that are not certified may contain gluten from other grains. This contamination can happen at any stage from field to grocery store shelf. The certification process ensures that gluten-free oats do not contain any gluten.

QUINOA SCRAMBLE

MAKES 2 SERVINGS

You can turn this simple scramble into a feast by serving it with muffins or millet rolls (page 73) and fresh fruit.

- 1 teaspoon olive oil (or less, if you use an olive oil spray)
- ½ cup onion, diced
- 1 cup sweet potatoes, peeled and diced
- ½ cup mushrooms, sliced
- 2 cups kale, deribbed and coarsely chopped
- 1 cup Basic Quinoa (page 18)
- ¼ to ½ teaspoon soy sauce, gluten-free tamari or coconut aminos (see note)

1. Heat olive oil in a large skillet over medium-high heat.
2. Add onion and sweet potatoes. Cook, stirring over medium-high heat, for 2 minutes.
3. Turn heat down to medium and add mushrooms. Sauté, stirring, for 1 minute.
4. Add kale, cooking another 2 minutes, or until kale is wilted.
5. Add quinoa and soy sauce (or tamari or coconut aminos), and stir until combined.
6. Remove from heat and serve.

NOTE: Tamari is a wheat-free soy sauce and is appropriate for people following a gluten-free diet. Coconut aminos is a soy-free sauce that has a zesty, salty flavor.

FRUIT-SWEETENED GRANOLA

MAKES 4 CUPS

As soon as you discover how easy it is to make your own granola, you may never buy packaged cereal again!

- 1 cup rolled oats (also called old-fashioned oats, gluten-free if necessary)
- 1 cup quinoa flakes
- ⅓ cup shelled pumpkin seeds (pepitas), finely chopped
- ¼ cup shelled hemp seeds
- ¼ cup apple juice
- ¼ cup date paste (see note)
- 2 tablespoons coconut oil, melted
- 1 teaspoon cinnamon
- ½ cup raisins or other dried fruit

1. Preheat oven to 350°F.
2. Combine oats, quinoa, seeds, apple juice, date paste, coconut oil, and cinnamon.
3. On a parchment-lined baking sheet, spread mixture in a thin layer.
4. Bake 15 to 20 minutes, or until golden brown.
5. When cool, combine mixture with raisins. Enjoy!

NOTE: To make your own date paste, pit and soak 6 Medjool dates for 15 minutes or more. Drain the softened dates and puree them in a blender. You can store date paste in a sealed container in the refrigerator for up to a week, or you can freeze it for up to 3 months.

VIBRANT YOGURT SMOOTHIE

MAKES 2 SERVINGS

You can prepare the beets for this delicious, gorgeously pink smoothie ahead of time. After you've cooked a batch, simply peel, chop, and freeze the beets until you're ready to use them. Watch out for the beet juice, though—it can stain your hands, clothes, dishtowels, and even your countertops. A little extra care is completely worth it, though, since beets are loaded with nutrition. They're a rich source of vitamins A, B, and C; folate; fiber; and minerals, including calcium and magnesium.

- *1 beet (see note)*
- *1 cup frozen strawberries*
- *1 teaspoon vanilla extract*
- *1 cup vanilla nondairy yogurt*
- *1 cup Hemp Milk (page 21) or other nondairy milk*
- *2 teaspoons chia seeds*
- *1 cup apple juice*

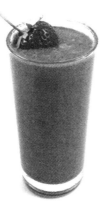

1. Wrap beet in foil and bake in a 400°F oven for 45 minutes. Let cool.

2. Remove beet skin and stem. Cut into chunks.

3. Combine all ingredients in blender. Blend until smooth.

NOTE: You can prebake beets, then refrigerate them for up to 3 days; if you cut them into chunks, they'll keep in the freezer for up to 3 months.

CH-CH-CH-CHIA

Many people first heard the word "chia" as a stuttered song in TV commercials for Chia Pets in the 1980s. These chia-covered clay figurines were wildly popular novelty gifts that originally came in the shape of rams and bulls. Today, Chia Pets are available in a wide range of shapes. And yes, those chia seeds are the same kind that will boost your health!

SUPERFOOD SMOOTHIE

MAKES 2 SERVINGS

Kale, blueberries, hemp, and chia seeds all in one tasty drink? That's getting your day off to a super start!

- *3 large kale leaves, deribbed and torn into pieces*
- *1 cup apple juice*
- *1 cup frozen mango chunks*
- *1 cup frozen blueberries*
- *1 cup Hemp Milk (page 21) or other nondairy milk*
- *2 tablespoons chia seeds*

1. In a blender, combine torn kale leaves and apple juice.
2. Blend on high until kale is completely broken down and liquefied.
3. Add remaining ingredients and blend until smooth.

SMOOTHIES MADE EASY

One way to always be ready for the next super-seed smoothie is to freeze hemp milk in ice cube trays, and then transfer the frozen cubes to a freezer-safe bag or container. When you want a smoothie, just blend some fruit with the frozen cubes and enjoy!

STRAWBERRY BREAKFAST PUDDING

MAKES 4 SERVINGS

Why not make breakfast a little more fun? Pudding for breakfast feels decadent, but with probiotic-rich yogurt, vitamin C–packed strawberries, and a protein boost from chia, this treat will power your morning.

- *2 six-ounce containers of strawberry-flavored nondairy yogurt*
- *½ cup applesauce*
- *½ cup strawberries (fresh or thawed frozen strawberries)*
- *2 tablespoons chia seeds (see note)*

1. Combine all ingredients in a blender or food processor. Blend thoroughly.
2. Divide pudding among four dessert dishes, small bowls, or coffee cups.
3. Cover and chill overnight.

NOTE: If you'd like a smoother pudding, grind the chia seeds in a clean grinder before adding them to the blender.

QUINOA BREAKFAST BURRITOS

MAKES 4 SERVINGS

Cholesterol-free quinoa stands in for eggs in this savory breakfast entree.

- 1 cup quinoa, rinsed
- 1 cup water
- 1 cup Basic Salsa (page 39), divided
- 4 whole-grain tortillas
- 1 avocado, cubed
- 1 large tomato, seeded and cubed
- ½ cup plain nondairy yogurt

1. In a small saucepan, combine quinoa, water, and ½ cup salsa. Bring to a boil.
2. Reduce heat, cover saucepan, and simmer for 15 minutes, or until germ ring spirals off the seed.
3. Heat tortillas, one at a time, in a dry skillet over high heat.
4. On a flat surface or plate, spoon about ½ cup quinoa onto each tortilla and top with a portion of avocado, tomato, salsa, and a dollop of yogurt.
5. Fold the bottom of the tortilla up, then roll it from one side to form a cylinder.

WAFFLES

MAKES 10

If you wrap these waffles individually, they'll keep in the freezer for up to a month. Then all you have to do is pop one into the toaster for a quick, warm breakfast.

- 3 tablespoons chia seeds
- ¾ cup water
- ¼ cup coconut oil, gently melted
- 2¼ cup Hemp Milk (page 21) or other nondairy milk
- 2 cups white whole-wheat flour
- 1 teaspoon salt
- 2 teaspoons baking powder

1. Combine chia seeds and water in a medium bowl and set aside for at least 10 minutes (to form gel).
2. Preheat waffle iron to medium-high.
3. Blend together chia gel, coconut oil, and hemp milk.
4. In a large bowl, whisk together flour, salt, and baking powder.
5. Mix in wet ingredients.
6. Pour ¼ cup mixture onto hot waffle iron.
7. Cook until golden brown, approximately 5 minutes.
8. Repeat with remaining batter.

COCONUT QUINOA GRANOLA

MAKES 3 CUPS

To make this granola nut-free you can use sunflower seeds, or shelled pumpkin seeds (pepitas) instead of almonds. Granolas are a great take-and-go snack that provide post-workout protein and healthy fats.

  1 cup quinoa flakes
  1 cup rolled oats (gluten-free if necessary)
  ¼ cup hulled hemp seeds
  ⅓ cup slivered almonds
  ½ cup unsweetened coconut flakes
  ⅛ teaspoon salt
  1 teaspoon cinnamon
  ¼ cup apple juice
  ¼ cup maple syrup

1. Preheat oven to 350°F.
2. In a large bowl, stir together all ingredients.
3. Spread the mixture in a thin, even layer on a large, rimmed parchment-lined baking sheet.
4. Bake for 15 minutes, stirring once half-way through, until granola is golden brown.
5. Place baking sheet on a wire rack and let granola cool completely before storing in an airtight container for up to 1 week.

CREAM OF AMARANTH

MAKES 1 SERVING

This is a delicious hot cereal that can be made nut-free by replacing the sliced almonds with toasted or raw hemp seeds.

  ½ cup Basic Amaranth (page 18)
  ¼ cup toasted almond slices (or ¼ cup shelled hemp seeds, toasted)
  ¼ cup raisins
  ¼ teaspoon cinnamon
  Hemp Milk (page 21) or other nondairy milk, warmed, to taste

1. Scoop warm, cooked amaranth into a cereal bowl.
2. Add almond slices (or toasted hemp seeds, if using) and raisins.
3. Sprinkle with cinnamon.
4. Top with warmed hemp milk, or other nondairy milk, and serve.

> ### WHAT ARE QUINOA FLAKES?
> Quinoa flakes are quinoa seeds that have been steam-rolled into flakes, giving them the appearance of rolled oats. In fact, you can substitute quinoa flakes for quick-cooking or old-fashioned rolled oats in many recipes, such as oatmeal cookies and granola. Quinoa flakes are gluten-free.

APRICOT QUINOA PORRIDGE

MAKES 2 SERVINGS

Quinoa makes a lovely hot cereal when you cook it in non-dairy milk instead of water or broth. You can also substitute fresh peaches for the dried apricots.

   ½ cup quinoa, rinsed
   1½ cups non-dairy milk
   1 tablespoon maple syrup
   ¼ cup chopped dried apricots

1. Combine all ingredients in a small saucepan.
2. Bring to a boil.
3. Cover and reduce heat. Simmer for 15 minutes.

SUMMER COOLER SMOOTHIE

MAKES 2 SERVINGS

If you are using mature spinach or kale for this smoothie, cut out any tough stems before blending. You can always use fresh rather than frozen fruit in this smoothie, but you might want to blend in a few ice cubes, as well.

   2 cups coconut water
   1 cup baby spinach or baby kale
   1 cup frozen pineapple
   1 cup frozen blueberries
   1 tablespoon chia seeds
   1 tablespoon ground flaxseed

1. Blend spinach or kale with coconut water until greens are broken down.
2. Add remaining ingredients and blend thoroughly.

WHAT IS THE DIFFERENCE BETWEEN COCONUT WATER AND COCONUT MILK?

Coconut water is a sweet-tasting transparent liquid that is collected from young coconuts. Many athletes promote drinking coconut water as a natural alternative to sports drinks because it contains potassium and sodium, which can promote rehydrating after a hard workout. Coconut milk is made from the flesh of mature coconuts. It is much higher in calories and fat than coconut water: One cup of full-fat coconut milk has 445 calories and 48 grams of fat (though light coconut milk is also available), while one cup of coconut water has 46 calories and no fat. A highly versatile ingredient, coconut milk can be used in a wide variety of cooked and raw dishes as well as baked goods and smoothies.

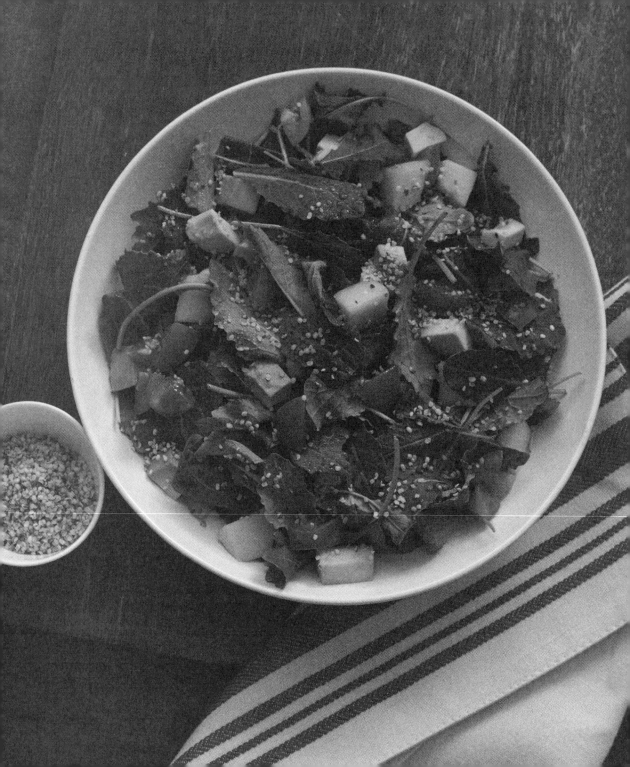

CHAPTER 4

SOUPS AND SALADS

S oups and salads are truly versatile—as light fare on their own or as a heartier meal when served together. And, if you want to bring a healthier, more substantial dish than the usual fatty, cholesterol-laden offering to a potluck (or to rustle up on the weekend or a busy weeknight), the recipes in this chapter will supply a tasty selection of alternatives that capitalize on the many nutritional benefits that super seeds deliver: iron, calcium, manganese, and a host of vitamins. They will fill you up, too, thanks to fiber-filled quinoa, amaranth, and hemp, but they won't weigh you down.

OPPOSITE: **Massaged Kale Salad, page 41**

LEMON BASIL QUINOA SALAD

MAKES 5 SERVINGS

Fresh lemon juice, basil, and capers give this hearty but light salad a bright Mediterranean flavor. It pairs beautifully with Pesto Veggie Burgers (page 62).

- 1 cup haricots verts (French green beans), trimmed and cut into ½-inch pieces
- 1 cup cucumbers, peeled, seeded, and cut into medium dice
- 2 cups Basic Quinoa (page 18)
- 10 cherry tomatoes, quartered
- 2 tablespoons plus 1 teaspoon capers, rinsed
- 2 tablespoons thinly sliced basil
- 1 tablespoon fresh lemon juice
- 1 tablespoon olive oil
  Salt and freshly ground black pepper

1. In a large bowl, toss all ingredients to combine.

QUINOA BLACK BEAN SALAD

SERVES 8

A quick and easy way to give quinoa, amaranth, or rice a deeper, more complex flavor is to add salsa, fresh lemon juice, soy sauce, or tamari (a gluten-free alternative to soy sauce) to the cooking water. This salad makes a terrific, light summer lunch.

- 1 cup quinoa, rinsed
- 1 cup Basic Salsa (page 39)
- 1 cup water
- 1 teaspoon salt
- 2 tomatoes, seeded and cut into small dice
- 1 cup corn kernels
- 1 avocado, cut into medium dice
- 1 15-ounce can black beans, drained and rinsed (or 1¾ cups cooked black beans)
- 1 tablespoon freshly squeezed lime juice
- 2 tablespoons cilantro, chopped

1. In a medium saucepan, combine quinoa, salsa, water, and salt. Bring to a boil. Cover, reduce heat, and simmer for 15 minutes.
2. In a large bowl, combine all ingredients. Serve chilled or at room temperature.

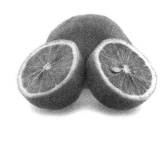

QUINOA LENTIL SOUP

MAKES APPROXIMATELY 10 SERVINGS

This filling, smoky-flavored soup is loaded with fiber and protein from both the lentils and the quinoa. If you are using thick carrots, cut them in half lengthwise before slicing them. Paired with a green salad, this makes a delicious and nutritious light supper or lunch.

1 *tablespoon olive oil*

2 *carrots, peeled and thinly sliced*

1 *onion, cut into small dice*

3 *cloves of garlic, minced*

1 *teaspoon ground cumin*

1 *teaspoon smoked paprika*

1 *15-ounce can tomato sauce or crushed tomatoes*

1 *cup dried red lentils, picked over and rinsed*

1 *cup quinoa, rinsed*

8 *cups water*

2 *teaspoons salt*

1. In a soup pot, heat olive oil over medium heat.

2. Add carrots and onion. Cook for 2 minutes, or until onion is softened.

3. Add garlic and cook for 1 more minute.

4. Add cumin and smoked paprika. Stir to distribute.

5. Add remaining ingredients. Bring to a boil.

6. Reduce heat to low, cover, and simmer 25 to 30 minutes, or until quinoa is cooked and lentils are soft.

ARE NUTRITIONAL YEAST AND BAKING YEAST THE SAME?

Nutritional yeast is a common ingredient in dairy-free cooking, because it has a savory, almost cheesy, flavor. It is a single-celled organism (*Saccharomyces Cerevisiae*) that is grown on molasses and then de-activated through drying. It is a good source of many nutrients, including many B vitamins – B_6, folate, and often B_{12} (which needs to be added to vegans' diets). It also is a good source of fiber, protein and zinc. Because nutritional yeast is deactivated, it won't help raise your bread dough, which relies on live yeast.

BLACK BEAN AND SWEET POTATO CHILI

MAKES 6 SERVINGS

This easy-to-prepare chili can warm up the coldest night. It's delicious served alongside a warm wedge of freshly baked Amaranth Cornbread (page 72). The tomatoes are also an excellent source of lycopene, an antioxidant that has been associated with prostate health—so serve it up with gusto the next time the guys come over to watch a game—or at any time, since this hearty chili is ideal for a quick, healthy meal.

  1 tablespoon olive oil

  3 medium onions, cut into medium dice (approximately 3 cups)

  3 medium garlic cloves, minced

  1 jalapeño pepper, ribs and seeds removed, minced

  1 medium sweet potato, peeled and cut into medium dice

  ¼ cup plus 2 tablespoons chili powder

  1 teaspoon ground cumin

  1 teaspoon dried oregano

  ½ teaspoon salt

  1 28-ounce can crushed tomatoes (3 cups)

  1 15-ounce can black beans, drained and rinsed (or 1¾ cups cooked black beans)

  1 cup Basic Quinoa (page 18)

1. In a large pot, heat olive oil over medium-high heat.

2. Add onions, garlic, jalapeño pepper, and sweet potato. Sauté approximately 5 minutes, or until vegetables are soft.

3. Add remaining ingredients, and bring to a boil.

4. Reduce heat and simmer for 20 to 25 minutes, or until heated through.

5. Serve with a warm wedge of Amaranth Cornbread.

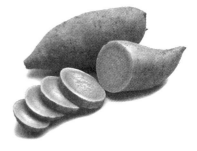

TACO SALAD

MAKES 4 SERVINGS

For this salad, I use canned mild chilies, because it suits my children's palate, but you can add more heat by substituting hotter canned peppers or dicing up a fresh jalapeno pepper.

- *2 cups vegetable broth*
- *2 tablespoons taco seasoning (see recipe on page 51)*
- *1 cup quinoa, rinsed and drained*
- *1 tablespoon olive oil*
- *1 cup chopped onion*
- *2 cups fresh, diced tomatoes*
- *1 cup chopped mild chilies, drained*
- *3 cups mixed lettuces*
- *1 medium red onion, chopped*
- *1 cup corn (either raw, cut from the cob, or defrosted frozen corn)*
- *½ cup black olives, sliced*
- *¼ cup fresh cilantro, chopped*
- *2 avocados, peeled and cut in ¾-inch chunks*
- *1 cup broken tortilla chips*
- *1 cup Basic Salsa (see recipe on page 39)*

1. In a small saucepan, bring vegetable broth, taco seasoning, and quinoa to a boil. Reduce heat, cover, and simmer for 15 minutes or until liquid is absorbed and the seeds look like little commas.

2. In a medium skillet, heat the olive oil over medium-high heat. Add onion, one cup diced tomato, and chilies. Sauté until soft. Add prepared quinoa to vegetables. Stir to combine.

3. In a large bowl, combine lettuces, remaining tomato, red onion, corn, black olives, and cilantro. Toss to mix. Divide lettuce mixture into four bowls or plates. Top with quinoa mixture. Add avocado. Top with tortilla chips and salsa to taste.

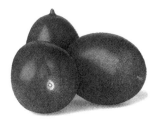

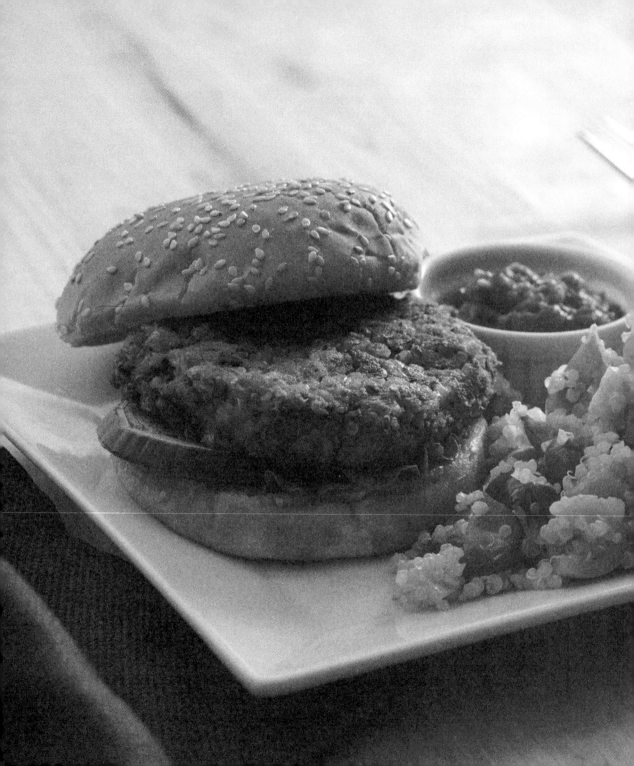

CHAPTER 5

ENTREES

The entrees in this chapter will not only satisfy your soul as you sit down to a family dinner or a holiday feast, they will also provide a good portion of the day's nutrition. With their broad nutrient profiles, chia, quinoa, flax, hemp, and amaranth contribute to dishes that are satisfying, nourishing, and delectable. With their rich load of plant-based protein and all nine essential amino acids, amaranth and quinoa elevate simple dishes like potato cakes and polenta, and fillings for stuffed avocados and squash, from supporting roles to the stars of well-rounded meals

OPPOSITE: **Pesto Veggie Burger with Lemon Basil Quinoa Salad, page 62**

TACO-SEASONED QUINOA-STUFFED AVOCADOS

MAKES 2 SERVINGS

At first it might seem odd to heat fresh, ripe avocados, but once you do, you'll be hooked: Just a little warming gives avocados' delicate flesh a super creamy, smooth consistency—perfect for this taco-flavored dish. If you don't want to use commercial taco seasoning, try my recipe below. I think you'll like it. And don't forget the tortilla chips for a nice, accompanying crunch!

- *1 teaspoon neutral-tasting oil (canola, grapeseed, or sunflower)*
- *¼ cup small-diced onion*
- *½ cup diced tomatoes (fresh or canned)*
- *1 tablespoon commercial taco seasoning (If using unsalted taco seasoning, add ½ teaspoon salt) or Kim's Basic Taco Seasoning (opposite)*
- *1 cup Basic Quinoa (page 18)*
- *1 ripe avocado*
- *2 lime wedges*

1. Preheat oven to 350°F.

2. In a medium skillet, heat oil over medium heat.

3. Add onion, tomatoes, and taco seasoning. Cook 2 to 3 minutes, or until onions are soft.

4. Add quinoa, stirring to combine. Remove from heat.

5. Halve avocado and remove pit. Scoop out avocado flesh with a spoon, leaving a ¼-inch border.

6. Chop flesh. Gently mix with filling.

7. Spoon half of the filling into the peel of an avocado half. Repeat with remaining filling.

8. Bake, filling-side up, for 10 to 12 minutes.

9. Remove from heat. Drizzle with fresh lime juice before serving.

TO MAKE THE STUFFING

1. Heat olive oil in a large skillet over medium heat.

2. Add onion and cook for 2 minutes, or until onions are soft but not brown.

3. Add apricots, paprika, cinnamon, and salt. Cook for 1 to 2 minutes.

4. Add almonds or pumpkin seeds, and stir to combine. Cook for another 2 minutes.

5. Remove mixture from heat and stir in amaranth. (If using amaranth that has been refrigerated, combine over heat for another 1 to 2 minutes.)

TO FINISH THE DISH

1. Scoop half of the filling into one of the squash halves.

2. Repeat with the other half of the squash.

3. Bake filling side up for 10 minutes.

4. Remove from oven and serve.

POTATO SCALLION PATTIES

MAKES 8 PATTIES

These crispy little fritters make a delicious light entree with a fresh green salad or roasted vegetables—they're also a great way to reuse leftover mashed potatoes.

> *3 medium baking potatoes, peeled and cubed*
>
> *1 cup Basic Amaranth (page 18)*
>
> *4 scallions, white and light green parts, thinly sliced*
>
> *2 teaspoons salt*
> *Freshly ground black pepper*
> *Olive oil spray*

1. In a large saucepan, cover potatoes with water and bring to a boil over medium heat.

2. Cook until potatoes are easily pierced with a fork.

3. Drain potatoes and place in a large bowl. Mash with a fork or a potato masher.

4. Add amaranth, scallions, and salt and pepper to potatoes. Mix well.

5. Lightly oil a skillet and heat until hot but not smoking.

6. Scoop out ¼ cup of potato mixture. Gently shape the mixture into a patty. Repeat with remaining mixture.

7. Sauté—in small batches so that they are not crowded in the skillet—for approximately 4 minutes per side, or until golden brown.

8. Keep patties warm in a 200–250 degree oven until all of them have been sautéed.

CAULIFLOWER HEMP CREAM LASAGNA

MAKES 6 SERVINGS

This lasagna is really satisfying. Depending on the texture you prefer, use a smooth tomato sauce for a silky lasagna or a chunky, vegetable-filled sauce for a heartier version. Gluten-free pasta can also be used, but what really makes this lasagna special is the cauliflower-hemp cream. Try pairing it with Massaged Kale Salad (page 41) for a complete meal.

3 cups pasta sauce of your choice

8 sheets of cooked whole-grain (or gluten-free) lasagna noodles (unless you are using "no-boil" pasta)

1 recipe Cauliflower Hemp Cream (recipe follows)

1. Preheat oven to 375°F.

2. Coat the bottom of a 9 × 13-inch baking dish with sauce.

3. Layer lasagna noodles on top of sauce, cover with cream, and repeat. Finish with sauce.

4. Bake, uncovered, for 40 minutes.

5. Remove from oven. Let stand 10 to 15 minutes before serving.

CAULIFLOWER HEMP CREAM

MAKES 4 CUPS

1 head cauliflower, stem discarded, chopped

2 tablespoons olive oil

1½ teaspoons kosher salt, divided

4 cloves garlic, peeled and smashed

½ teaspoon freshly ground black pepper

2 tablespoons nutritional yeast

½ teaspoon dry mustard

1 cup Hemp Milk (page 21)

1. Preheat oven to 425°F.

2. Toss together cauliflower, olive oil, 1 teaspoon salt, and garlic, then spread cauliflower on an ungreased baking sheet or a baking sheet lined with parchment paper.

3. Bake 20 minutes, or until cauliflower is tender.

4. Puree cauliflower with remaining ingredients, including remaining salt.

NOTE: You can use this savory cream as a topping for steamed vegetables and baked potatoes, or toss it with your favorite pasta. Store any extra cauliflower cream in a sealed container in the refrigerator for up to 3 days.

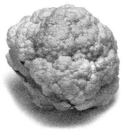

AMARANTH POLENTA
WITH SAUTÉED MUSHROOMS

MAKES 6 SERVINGS

Polenta is a true comfort food that can easily be converted into a complete, protein-rich meal by adding amaranth and hemp milk to the cornmeal. Sautéed Mushrooms (recipe follows) beautifully complement the creamy texture of the polenta, but feel free to experiment with other toppings such as pasta sauce, sautéed greens, or anything else you can think of.

AMARANTH POLENTA

    3 cups Hemp Milk (page 21)
    ½ teaspoon salt
    ½ cup amaranth flour
    ½ cup medium- or coarsely ground cornmeal
    1 cup water
    ¼ teaspoon freshly ground black pepper

1. Bring hemp milk and salt to a boil.
2. Whisk in amaranth, cornmeal, and pepper; reduce heat to a simmer.
3. Add water. Stir to thoroughly combine.
4. Cook for 30 to 45 minutes, stirring the mixture regularly until it is very thick.
5. Keep polenta warm until ready to serve.

SAUTÉED MUSHROOMS

    2 tablespoons olive oil
    1 teaspoon dried oregano
    1 teaspoon dried thyme
    ¼ cup diced onion
    8 ounces cremini mushrooms, sliced
        (approximately 3 cups)
    1 medium tomato, diced (approximately
        1 cup)
    ½ teaspoon salt
    ¼ teaspoon freshly ground black pepper
    2 tablespoons fresh basil leaves, thinly sliced

1. In a large skillet over medium heat, heat oil and sauté oregano and thyme till the herbs give off their aromas.
2. Add onions, then sauté 2 to 3 minutes, or until onions are soft.
3. Add mushrooms, tomato, and salt and pepper. Cook, stirring over medium heat for 2 to 3 minutes, or until mushrooms are soft.
4. Transfer mushroom mixture to a serving bowl.
5. Dress each portion of warm polenta with a generous scoop of sautéed mushrooms and garnish with basil. Serve in warm bowls and enjoy.

BARBECUE BEANS

SERVES 4

This recipe gives you the slow-cooked flavor and texture of baked beans without the wait. Pureed sweet potato adds creaminess and sweet flavor, while a mere two tablespoons of chia transform the sauce into syrupy goodness. For a complete meal, serve these awesome beans with a thick slice of warm Whole-Grain Spelt and Amaranth Loaf (page 62) or a Whole-Grain Millet Roll (page 73) fresh from the oven. Don't forget the green salad!

- 1 tablespoon olive oil
- 1 cup onion, cut in small dice
- ½ cup pureed sweet potato
- 2 tablespoons chia seeds
- ½ cup barbecue sauce
- 1 15-ounce can canellini beans, drained and rinsed

1. In a sauté pan, heat oil over medium heat.
2. Add onion. Cook until soft.
3. Add remaining ingredients and cook until heated through.
4. Let beans rest for at least 15 minutes and stir before serving.

WHITE CHIA
VS. BLACK CHIA

Chia seeds—white and black—are multipurpose stars in the kitchen with a very subtle flavor. There is no significant nutritional difference between white and black chia, although white seeds are more rare than black seeds and cost a bit more because of their rarity. Black or white, chia seeds have been touted as one of the most nutrient-dense foods available today, and they are used in myriad ways—to boost energy, assist in weight loss, and help regulate blood sugar. For the recipes in this book, there is no need to go out of your way to buy one color chia seed or the other—they'll turn out just fine no matter which chia seed you use.

EASY BARBECUE SAUCE

MAKES 1 CUP

This barbecue sauce is smoky-sweet, with just the right amount of heat. You can play with the flavor by experimenting with strawberry or even blueberry jelly or preserves instead of using grape jelly or preserves.

> ½ *chipotle pepper in adobo sauce, minced*
> 1 *15-ounce can tomato sauce*
> 2 *tablespoons all-fruit grape jelly or preserves*
> 2 *tablespoons apple cider vinegar*

1. In a small saucepan over medium heat, combine all ingredients and bring to a boil.
2. Reduce heat and simmer uncovered for 30 minutes. The sauce should be thick and reduced by about half.
3. Use immediately or store in the refrigerator in a tight-lidded container for up to 1 week.

CHAI-SPICED SWEET POTATO

SERVES 1

Sweet potatoes are excellent sources of Vitamins A and C. They are loaded with fiber and, surprisingly, they are not overly high in calories, despite their sweetness and rich texture. One large sweet potato averages only about 160 calories, making this unusual spiced tea–inflected recipe a filling, flavorful lunch that won't expand your waistline.

> 1 *baked sweet potato*
> 1 *to 3 tablespoons brewed spiced tea, such as chai*
> 2 *to 4 tablespoons shelled hemp seeds*
> *salt to taste*

1. Scoop flesh from sweet potato and mash with a fork.
2. Gradually stir a little tea into the mashed sweet potato, until you have achieved the texture you desire.
3. In a dry skillet, toast hemp seeds over medium heat for 30 seconds or so, until fragrant but not burned.
4. Sprinkle hemp seeds and salt over the warm, mashed sweet potato and enjoy.

VEGGIE "MEATBALLS"

MAKES 40 BALLS

Commercial, frozen veggie meatballs can be filled with processed ingredients, but if you make your own, you can control what goes into the mix. You can also change up the flavor according to your preferences. Different spices, for example, can provide a different flavor profile altogether. Enjoy them in a sandwich, served with pasta, or all on their own! They are *so* good.

- 2 cups Rich Soup Base (opposite), vegetable broth, or water
- ½ teaspoon salt
- 1 cup kasha (roasted buckwheat)
- ¼ cup flaxseed meal
- ½ cup water
- 8 ounces button or cremini mushrooms
- 6 sundried tomato halves, softened in hot water
- 2 tablespoons olive oil, divided
- 1 15-ounce can garbanzo beans, drained and rinsed (or 1¾ cups cooked)
- 1 large or 2 small cloves garlic, smashed
- 1 teaspoon dried rosemary
- 1 teaspoon dried oregano
- 1 teaspoon dried thyme
- Freshly ground black pepper

1. In a small saucepan, bring soup base (or broth or water) and salt to a boil.

2. Add kasha, reduce heat, cover, and simmer for 10 minutes, or until liquid is absorbed. Set aside.

3. In a small bowl, thoroughly mix together flaxseed meal and water. Set aside.

4. In a food processor, finely chop mushrooms and drained tomatoes.

5. Heat 2 teaspoons of olive oil in a skillet. Add mushrooms and tomatoes. Cook until liquid released from the mushrooms has cooked down.

6. While mushrooms are cooking, blend chickpeas and garlic into a paste.

7. In a large bowl, mix all components together, adding the herbs and freshly ground black pepper.

8. Chill mixture in the refrigerator for 30 minutes.

9. Preheat oven to 375°F.

10. Prep two baking sheets with remaining olive oil.

11. Roll meatball mixture into 1½-inch balls and place meatballs on prepared baking sheets.

12. Bake for 30 minutes, or until browned.

13. Let the meatballs stand for a few minutes before serving, since they will be fragile when first removed from the oven.

14. Serve in warm sauce or gravy.

RICH SOUP BASE

YIELD = 6–7 CUPS

Instead of using vegetable broth in your recipes, consider using a rich homemade soup base that will increase the fiber and nutrients in your food. It's easy to do: Just prepare a basic vegetable soup and put it through the blender to get a rich broth or base for recipes such as Veggie "Meatballs" (opposite). You can cook up a big pot, either on the stove or in a slow cooker, and freeze it in 1- or 2-cup portions to use whenever you need a soup starter, a liquid for macaroni and cheese, or to enrich another sauce. I stay away from starchy vegetables, such as potatoes and corn, because they will make the soup base too creamy for some uses. You can make as much of this soup base as you like, depending on the size of your soup pot and the quantity of vegetables you use.

4 cups carrots, onions, garlic, kale (or any other combination of veggies, depending on what you have on hand)

Water

Salt and freshly ground black pepper, to taste

1. Wash and roughly chop all vegetables.

2. Put vegetables in a stockpot and cover with water. (Tops of vegetables should be covered with at least 3 inches of water.)

3. Bring to a boil, cover stockpot, and reduce heat. Simmer for 30 to 40 minutes, or until vegetables are tender.

4. Transfer mixture, in batches, to a blender and blend thoroughly.

DECONSTRUCTED BROCCOLI SOUP CASSEROLE

MAKES 6 SERVINGS

In this recipe, I've combined two things that my family loves—broccoli cheese soup and casseroles. Cashew Hemp "Cheese" Sauce (opposite) gives this dish its rich, satisfying texture. For a nut-free version, substitute Cauliflower Hemp Cream (page 54).

1 teaspoon olive oil

3 cups thinly sliced baking potatoes (russet, red, or gold)

¼ teaspoon salt, divided

½ cup diced onions

3 cups broccoli, chopped in small pieces

¼ teaspoon salt, divided

1½ cups Cashew Hemp "Cheese" Sauce or nut-free Cauliflower Hemp Cream.

1. Preheat oven to 375°F.
2. Spread olive oil over the bottom of a 9 × 13-inch baking pan.
3. Cover the bottom of the pan with a single layer of potatoes.
4. Sprinkle potatoes with ⅛ teaspoon salt.
5. Spoon half of the onions then half of the broccoli over the potatoes.
6. Pour half of the cheese sauce over the onions and broccoli.
7. Repeat with remaining ingredients.
8. Bake for 45 minutes, or until potatoes are cooked through and there is bubbling around the edges.

SUMMERY (SUPER SEED) LINEN

When the temperature rises, linen dresses and slacks appear in the pages of clothing catalogues and shop windows. Why? Because linen, a fabric made from flax, keeps you feeling cool even as things are heating up.

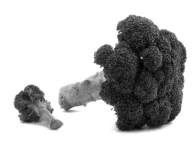

CASHEW HEMP "CHEESE" SAUCE

MAKES 1½ CUPS

You can toss whole-grain pasta, quinoa, or vegetables with this nutrient-rich, cheesy sauce, or use it as the base for a comforting entrée, such as Deconstructed Broccoli Soup Casserole (opposite).

> *1 cup raw unsalted cashews, soaked for 4 to 6 hours or overnight and drained and rinsed*
>
> *¼ cup hemp seeds*
>
> *2 tablespoons apple cider vinegar*
>
> *1 teaspoon salt*
>
> *2 tablespoons nutritional yeast*
>
> *½ teaspoon smoked paprika*
>
> *1 cup unsweetened Hemp Milk (page 21) or other nondairy milk*

1. In a blender, process all ingredients until smooth.

2. Pour mixture into a small saucepan.

3. Cook over medium heat, stirring occasionally, 5 to 8 minutes, or until gently bubbling.

4. Remove from heat, toss with pasta, grain, or veggies of your choice, and serve. Yum.

5. You can add extra hemp milk to thin to desired consistency.

NUTTY SANDWICH SPREAD

MAKES 1½ CUPS

This savory sandwich spread is equally satisfying spread on a crusty roll, smeared into a fresh lettuce wrap, or served as a dip with an array of crunchy vegetables.

> *1 cup cashews, soaked for at least 4 hours in fresh water, then drained*
>
> *½ cup hemp seed*
>
> *½ teaspoon salt*
>
> *½ tablespoon prepared Dijon mustard*
>
> *4 sundried tomato halves, cut into small dice*

1. Blend all ingredients in a food processor until smooth.

2. Transfer the mixture to a small saucepan and cook over medium heat for 5 minutes, stirring to keep mixture from burning.

3. Cool and store spread in a covered container in the refrigerator for up to 1 week.

PESTO VEGGIE BURGERS

MAKES 4 PATTIES

To give these hearty veggie burgers a bolder flavor, feel free to add more pesto to the mix. The burgers are delicious on a seeded bun with a slice of red onion and a couple of crisp leaves of lettuce. Lemon Basil Quinoa Salad (page 38) makes a perfect partner.

1 tablespoon flaxseed meal

3 tablespoons water

1 tablespoon olive oil

1 tablespoon minced shallots

1 cup cremini mushrooms, cut into small dice

1 15-ounce can cannellini beans, drained and rinsed

1 tablespoon Hemp Pesto (page 21)

½ cup quinoa flakes

Salt and freshly ground black pepper, to taste

Olive oil spray

1. In a small bowl, combine flaxseed meal and water. Set aside.

2. In a medium skillet, heat olive oil over medium heat.

3. Add shallots and mushrooms and cook for 2 to 3 minutes, or until vegetables are softened.

4. In a large bowl, combine flaxseed meal and cannellini beans. Mash with a potato masher.

5. Add the mushroom mixture, hemp pesto, quinoa flakes, and salt and pepper to the bowl, mixing together.

6. Shape mixture into 4 patties.

7. Spray a medium skillet with olive oil.

8. Over medium heat, cook patties, 4 to 5 minutes per side, until they are warm all the way through.

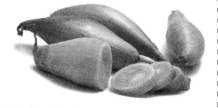

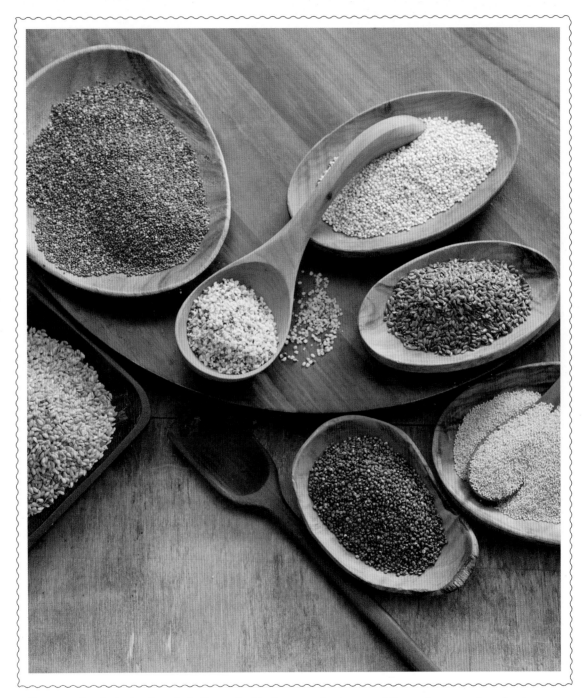

Super seeds, clockwise from left: flaxseed, chia, hemp, quinoa, roasted flaxseed, amaranth, red quinoa

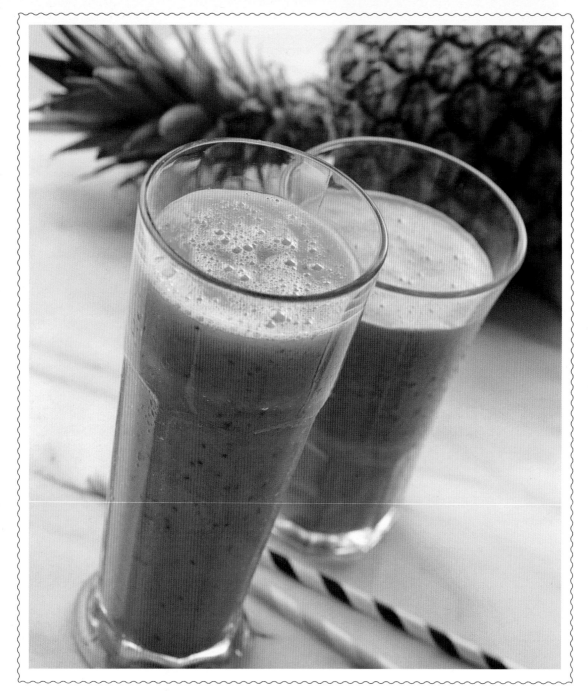

Foreground: Carrot Sweet Potato Yogurt Smoothie, page 27; Background: Vibrant Yogurt Smoothie, page 31

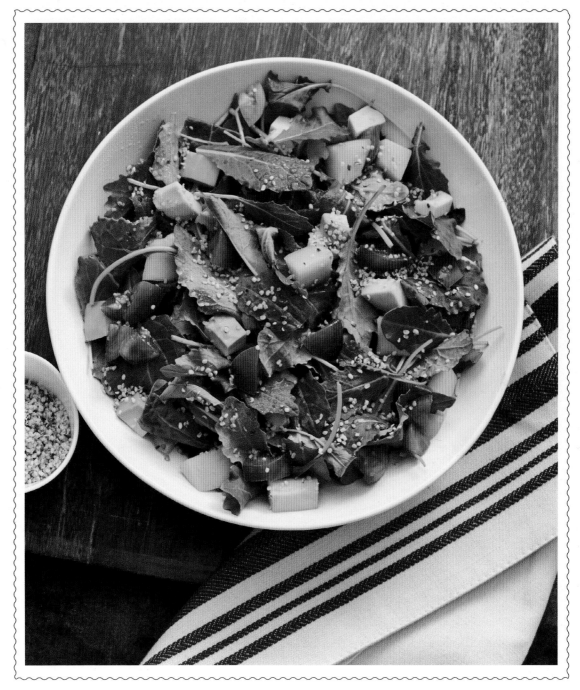

Massaged Kale Salad, page 41

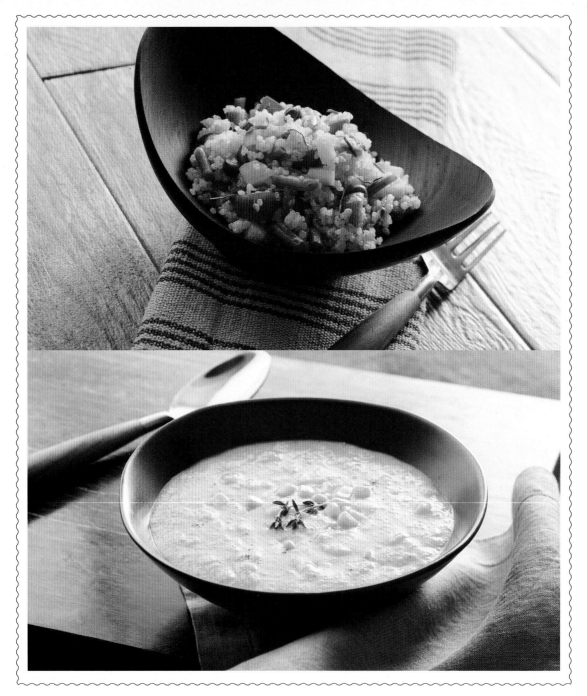

TOP: Lemon Basil Quinoa Salad, page 38; BOTTOM: Golden Corn Soup, page 43

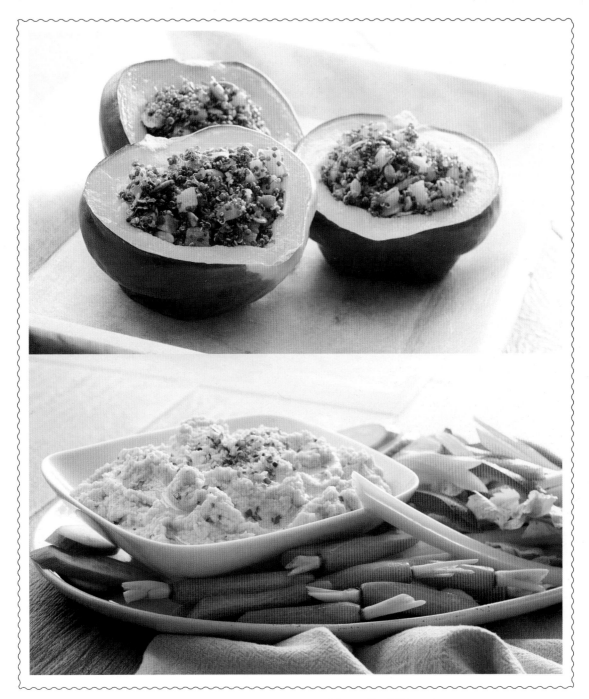

TOP: Amaranth-Stuffed Acorn Squash, page 52; BOTTOM: Hemp Seed Hummus, page 64

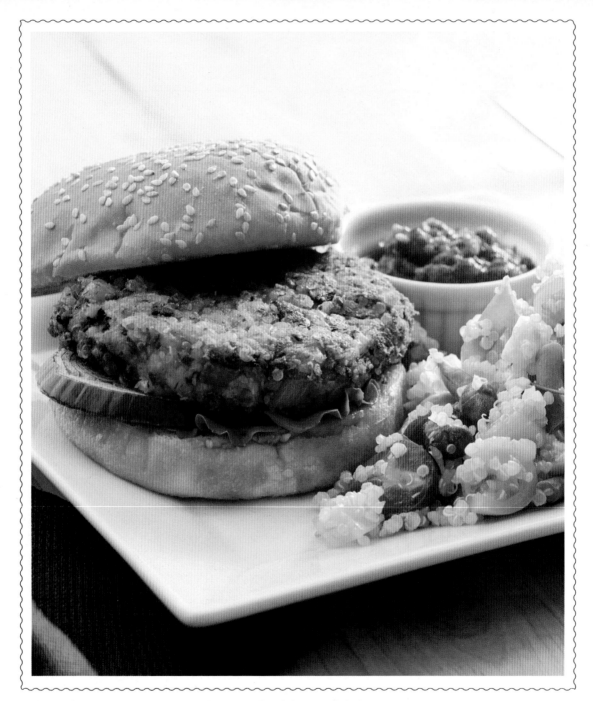

Pesto Veggie Burger, page 62, with Lemon Basil Quinoa Salad, page 38

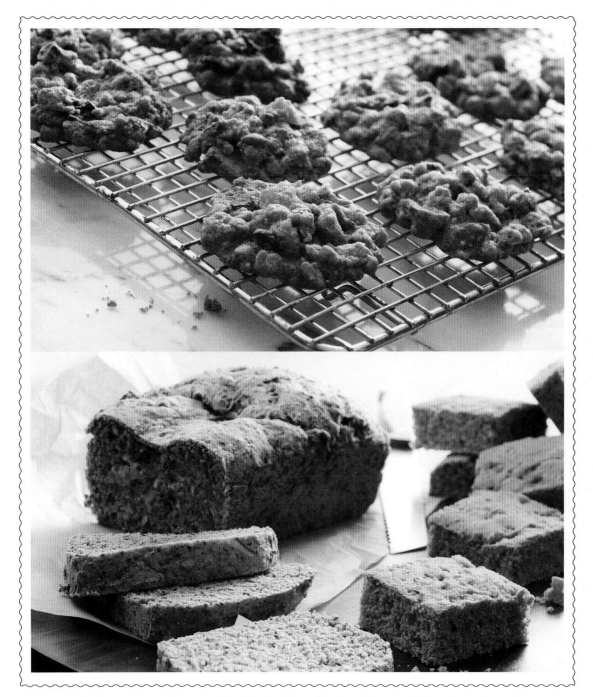

Granola Cookies, page 97; Bottom, left: Whole-Grain Spelt and Amaranth Loaf, page 70; right: Amaranth Cornbread, page 72

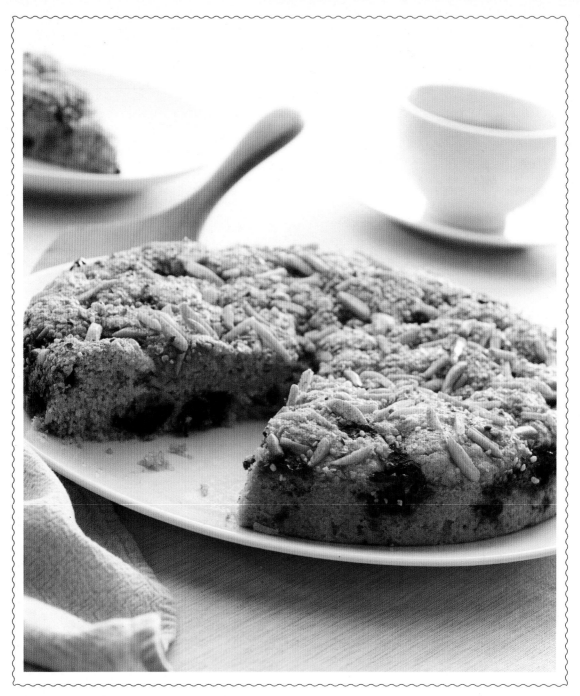

Blueberry Coffee Cake, page 78

ENCHILADA CASSEROLE

MAKES 4 GENEROUS SERVINGS

If you're craving tacos instead of a casserole, simply prepare the filling for these enchiladas and scoop it into either crunchy or soft tortillas. Then lay out a spread of toppings—shredded lettuce or cabbage, chopped tomatoes, onions, guacamole (or sliced avocado), and extra salsa—and enjoy the feast! (To keep this dish gluten-free, use gluten-free taco shells or tortillas.)

> 1 15-ounce can crushed tomatoes
>
> 2 tablespoons commercial taco seasoning or Kim's Basic Taco Seasoning (page 51)
>
> 1 15-ounce can black beans, rinsed (or 1½ cups cooked black beans)
>
> 1½ cups Basic Amaranth (page 18)
>
> 1 cup diced red bell pepper
>
> 1 cup corn kernels
>
> 1½ cups prepared salsa or Basic Salsa (page 39)
>
> 8 10-inch tortillas (whole-grain or gluten-free)

1. Preheat oven to 375°F.

2. In a large bowl, combine tomatoes with taco seasoning.

3. Add beans, amaranth, red pepper, and corn. Stir to combine.

4. Spoon ½ cup salsa onto bottom of a 9 × 13-inch baking pan or casserole dish.

5. Place one tortilla on a plate. Spoon ⅛ of the mixture onto the left side of the tortilla, leaving a 1- to 2-inch margin. Roll the tortilla and filling into a tube and place rolled tortilla into dish.

6. Continue with remaining tortillas, laying them next to each other until they tightly fill the pan.

7. Spread remaining salsa over enchiladas.

8. Bake for 35 to 40 minutes. There will be bubbling around the edges of the pan when it's done.

A TIME AND MONEY SAVER

You can save money by buying ingredients—cashews and almonds, for example—from bulk bins at your local grocery or health food store, and also save time by soaking them overnight and then freezing the soaked (and drained) nuts until you need them. All you have to do is thaw them and you're ready to cook!

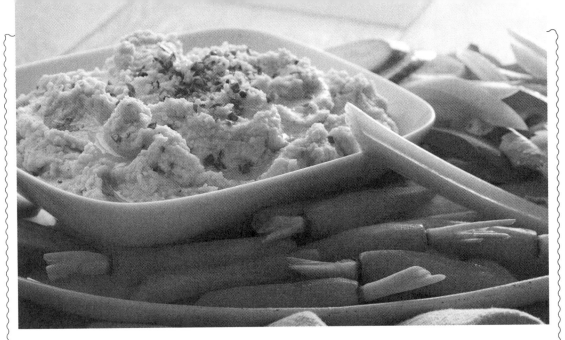

HEMP SEED HUMMUS

MAKES 1½ CUPS

Hemp seeds do double duty in this recipe. First, they take the place of the traditional ingredient in hummus, tahini (some people are allergic to sesame seeds). Second, they bring crucial phytonutrients, including zinc and magnesium, to this tasty, satisfyingly textured dip. It makes a great snack, served with crudités such as baby carrots, cucumber slices, celery sticks, and strips of crunchy bell peppers. In addition to making superb sandwiches, hummus is also a salad's best friend. Try adding a healthy dollop on top of your green salad and you will have a flavorful, filling meal.

1¾ cups cooked garbanzo beans (or one 15-ounce can, drained and rinsed)

2 tablespoons hemp seeds

2 tablespoons lemon juice

¼ teaspoon ground cumin

½ teaspoon salt

3 tablespoons olive oil

1 clove garlic, minced

2 tablespoons water

1. Blend all ingredients together in a food processor or blender until smooth.

PINEAPPLE FRIED QUINOA

MAKES 4 SIDE-DISH SERVINGS
OR 2 MAIN-DISH SERVINGS

This spicy-sweet one-dish meal featuring fiber- and protein-rich quinoa comes together quickly. Delicious!

- 3 tablespoons soy sauce, gluten-free tamari or coconut aminos
- ¼ cup fresh orange juice
- ¼ teaspoon sriracha hot sauce
- 2 teaspoons neutral-tasting oil (canola, grapeseed, or sunflower)
- 2 cloves garlic, minced
- 2 carrots, peeled, halved, and thinly sliced
- 1 cup sliced mushrooms (button, cremini, or shitake)
- 1 cup diced pineapple, fresh or thawed
- 2½ cups broccoli florets and peeled, chopped stems
- 2 cups Basic Quinoa (page 18)

1. In a small bowl, combine soy sauce or tamari or coconut aminos, orange juice, and sriracha. Set aside.

2. In a large skillet, heat oil over medium-high heat.

3. Add garlic, carrots, and mushrooms. Cook, stirring, for 2 minutes.

4. Add pineapple and broccoli. Cook for another 2 minutes, or until broccoli is bright green.

5. Add sauce to the mixture in the skillet and combine.

6. Add quinoa and cook until the mixture is warmed through. Serve immediately.

HEMP TOFU LASAGNA

SERVES 4

Blending hemp tofu with non-dairy milk makes a delicious alternative to ricotta cheese. If you don't have lasagna noodles on hand, you can layer almost any other form of cooked pasta with layers of sauce and filling; it tastes just as good.

1 8-ounce package of hemp tofu

1 cup hemp or other non-dairy milk

¼ cup basil leaves

2 cups spinach leaves, tough stems removed

4 artichoke hearts

2 tablespoons nutritional yeast

1 tablespoon garlic pepper

2 cups pasta sauce

10–12 whole grain lasagna noodles (no-boil or prepared)

¼ cup vegan mozzarella cheese shreds (optional)

1. Preheat oven to 375.

2. In a food processor, thoroughly blend together tofu and non-dairy milk.

3. Add basil, spinach, artichoke hearts, nutritional yeast, and garlic pepper. Process until smooth.

4. Spread ⅓ of the pasta sauce in the bottom of a lasagna pan or 9 × 13 baking dish.

5. Lay noodles on top of sauce in a single layer.

6. Spread half of the tofu mixture on top of the noodles.

7. Layer sauce, noodles, and tofu on top of that.

8. Top with remaining noodles and sauce.

9. Sprinkle with cheese if, using.

10. Bake for 40 minutes or until bubbly.

HEMP TOFU—A DELICIOUS SOY-FREE ALTERNATIVE

Even if you can't have soy, you can still enjoy tofu. Tempt Living Foods is marketing a hemp-based tofu in the United States. Not only is tofu a tasty addition to stir-fries and Asian soups, it can also be crumbled and blended with other ingredients to create luscious lasagnas, savory bread puddings, and quiches.

QUICK AND CHUNKY PASTA SAUCE

SERVES 4

1 tablespoon olive oil
1 large clove garlic (or 2 small cloves)
1 teaspoon dried basil
1 teaspoon dried oregano
½ teaspoon dried thyme
1 28-ounce can diced tomatoes, drained
    salt and pepper to taste

1. In a medium saucepan, heat olive oil over medium heat.
2. Smash and mince garlic, add to olive oil.
3. Cook for 30 seconds, add dried spices and stir. Cook for another 30 seconds or so.
4. Add drained tomatoes, stir to combine, and simmer for 10 minutes (or longer, if you have time).

MIDDLE EASTERN–INSPIRED LENTILS AND QUINOA

MAKES 6 SERVINGS

I serve this dish with a green salad for a quick, but satisfying weeknight dinner.

1 cup quinoa, rinsed
4¼ cups vegetable broth
1 cup brown lentils, rinsed and picked over
½ teaspoon cumin
1 teaspoon salt
2 tablespoons olive oil
1 cup chopped onion
1 cup chopped carrot
    freshly ground black pepper, to taste

1. In a large saucepan, combine quinoa, vegetable broth, lentils, cumin, and salt.
2. Bring to a boil. Reduce heat, cover pan, and simmer on low heat for 30 minutes, or until lentils are tender.
3. While the quinoa is cooking, heat olive oil over high heat.
4. Fry the onion and carrots until golden brown.
5. Fluff quinoa and lentils; serve on a platter topped with onions and freshly ground pepper.

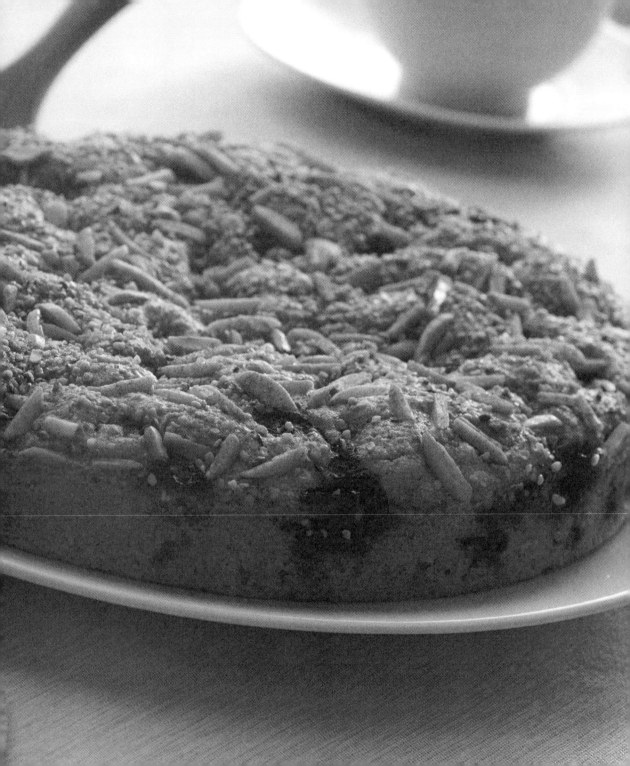

CHAPTER 6

BAKED GOODS

The recipes in this chapter celebrate a range of delicious treats from muffins, rolls, and breads to decadent breakfast cakes that capitalize on the unique flavors, textures, and aromas of super seeds such as flaxseed and chia, combined with the richness of fresh produce such as pumpkin and zucchini, and market-fresh berries, apples, and pears. You'll even find super seed and chocolate combos that will quickly motivate you to tie on your apron and warm up the oven. You'll be surprised by how easy it is (and how great it tastes) to bake with super seed flours such as amaranth and flaxseed meal, along with whole-grain spelt, millet, and whole-wheat or gluten-free oat flour. Give it a shot and be prepared to change the way you bake!

OPPOSITE: **Blueberry Coffee Cake, page 78**

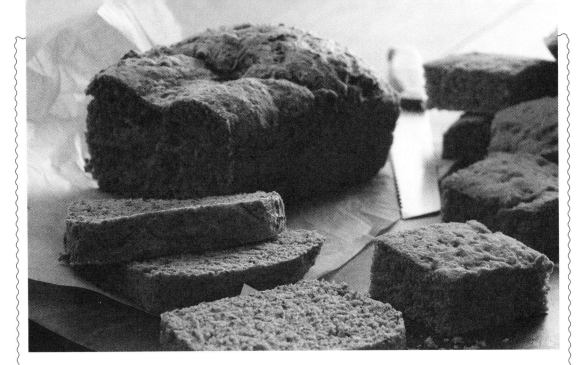

WHOLE-GRAIN SPELT AND AMARANTH LOAF

MAKES ONE STANDARD BREAD LOAF

This whole-grain loaf bakes up golden and aromatic. Sliced, it is ideal for toasty sandwiches.

1½ cups warm water
1½ teaspoons active dry yeast
1½ teaspoons salt
2 cups whole-grain spelt
1¼ cups amaranth flour

1. In a large bowl, combine water and yeast.
2. Add remaining ingredients and stir to thoroughly combine.
3. Cover the bowl and set it in a warm spot for 1½ to 2 hours, or until the dough has doubled in size.
4. Preheat oven to 425°F.
5. Lightly oil a standard bread pan.
6. Scoop dough into the prepared pan, lightly smoothing the top with damp hands.
7. Bake for 35 minutes. You'll know the bread is done when it's golden brown and, when you remove the loaf from the pan, the bottom sounds hollow when you tap it with your knuckles.
8. Remove the bread from the oven and turn out the loaf onto a rack or a clean kitchen towel. Allow to cool before slicing.

THE EASY WAY
TO MAKE YOUR OWN FLOUR

Buying a good-quality nut or spice grinder can pay for itself many times over if you use seed flours and nut butters as much as I do. For example, you can purchase a bag of rolled oats or buy them in bulk and easily grind up all the oat flour you need for a batch of muffins or cookies. If you need amaranth flour and have only whole amaranth on hand, your nut grinder can step in beautifully to supply what you need. If you don't have a spice or nut grinder, you can use your electric coffee grinder. To keep it clean between uses, just grind up a piece of plain bread. What could be easier?

* * *

FEAR OF KNEADING

If you've been reluctant to bake your own bread because kneading and working with yeast sounds tricky, spelt flour was made for you! Spelt truly is a wonder grain, not the least because it requires *no* kneading to bake beautifully. It contains a broad spectrum of vitamins, such as B2 and nutrients, including complex carbs, fiber, minerals, amino acids, and a lot more. To bake with spelt flour, all you need to do is mix it in with the other ingredients in your recipe, let the dough rise, and then either shape it into rolls or scoop the dough into a loaf pan and bake it. The air pockets that form during the first rise will give your bread a lovely texture—without any hassles.

AMARANTH CORNBREAD

MAKES 9 SERVINGS

This delicious quick bread, the perfect accompaniment to chili, beautifully pairs amaranth and corn while supplying plenty of protein, fiber, and phytonutrients, too.

- ¾ cup cornmeal
- ½ cup amaranth flour
- ¾ cup white whole-wheat flour
- ½ teaspoon evaporated cane juice or coconut palm sugar
- 2¼ teaspoons baking powder, divided
- 1 teaspoon baking soda
- ½ teaspoon salt
- ¼ cup applesauce
- 3 tablespoons neutral-tasting oil (canola, grapeseed, or sunflower)
- 1 cup Hemp Milk (page 21) or other nondairy milk

1. Preheat oven to 400°F.

2. In a medium bowl, combine cornmeal, flours, sweetener, 2 teaspoons baking powder, baking soda, and salt with a whisk.

3. In a large bowl, combine applesauce with ¼ teaspoon baking powder.

4. Add oil and nondairy milk to applesauce mixture.

5. Mix dry ingredients into wet ingredients.

6. Pour the mixture into an 8-inch-square baking pan that has been coated with oil or lined with parchment paper.

7. Bake for 20 minutes, or until a toothpick inserted in the middle of the bread comes out clean. Cut into squares and serve.

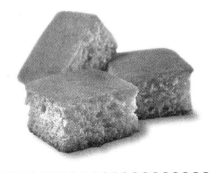

WHOLE-GRAIN MILLET ROLLS

MAKES 8

When you serve these homey rolls with a good bowl of soup, you'll enjoy a warm and soul-satisfying meal. Millet, a tiny, ancient grain, is a good source of manganese, phosphorus, and magnesium.

1½ cups warm water

1 package rapid rise yeast

2 teaspoons salt

1 tablespoon maple syrup

2 cups whole-grain spelt flour

½ cup flaxseed meal

¼ cup millet

1 tablespoon olive oil

1. In a large bowl, combine water, yeast, salt, and maple syrup. Let the mixture sit for 10 minutes.

2. Mix in spelt, flaxseed meal, and millet.

3. Coat the dough with olive oil.

4. Place the dough in a large bowl and cover it.

5. Keep the bowl in a warm place for 1½ hours or until dough has doubled.

6. Preheat oven to 425°F.

7. Lightly shape dough into dinner rolls.

8. Place the rolls on a parchment paper–covered baking pan.

9. Bake 15 to 18 minutes. Rolls are done when they sound hollow when tapped on the bottom.

10. Place on a cooling rack.

IS SPELT A FORM OF WHEAT?

If you're confused about spelt's family tree, there's a reason why! Although spelt is an ancient grain, it is in the wheat family, and it contains gluten, similar to wheat. If spelt isn't as well known or as widely used as wheat, there's a reason for that, too. Spelt simply has not had the same history of hybridization and cross-breeding that modern wheat has enjoyed, despite the fact that spelt has been grown for hundreds of years in Europe, and possibly thousands of years before that in the Middle East. Some people claim that spelt is easier to digest than wheat, but if you have celiac disease or a wheat allergy, avoid spelt.

AMARANTH BISCUITS

MAKES 8

When you slice these biscuits in half lengthwise, they make a great sandwich roll, and, because they are made with cooked amaranth and nondairy yogurt, instead of butter, margarine, or shortening, they are not loaded with saturated fat and cholesterol. Turn these biscuits into a satisfying sandwich by spreading with Hemp Seed Hummus (page 64) and adding some tomato and cucumber slices.

> 1 cup white whole-wheat flour
> 1 teaspoon baking powder
> ½ teaspoon baking soda
> ¼ teaspoon salt
> ½ cup Basic Amaranth (page 18)
> 1 cup plain nondairy yogurt

1. Preheat oven to 425°F.

2. In a large bowl, whisk together flour, baking powder, baking soda, and salt.

3. Mix in amaranth and yogurt. Stir to combine.

4. Spoon batter onto a baking sheet lined with parchment paper.

5. Bake for 12 to 15 minutes, or until golden brown.

6. Remove from oven and place biscuits on a cooling rack.

DOES EVERYTHING HAVE TO BE "ORGANIC"?

When you're trying to eat healthier, one of the factors to consider is whether you should always buy organic produce or whether it's okay to buy conventionally grown produce. Eating fruits and vegetables is a key component to a healthy diet, but pesticide residue can be a problem. How do you know which veggies and fruit should always be bought organic and which are okay to eat without that designation? Luckily, the Environmental Working Group (EWG) examines the pesticide residues on a wide range of produce and publishes an annual guide to what should always be purchased organic, "The Dirty Dozen," and what can be bought conventional, "The Clean Fifteen." To find out which is which, visit www.ewg.org.

ZUCCHINI BREAD OR MUFFINS

MAKES 2 LOAVES OR 18 MUFFINS

This is a versatile recipe that yields sweet treats that can travel from the breakfast table to the dessert plate by adding a cup of chocolate chips to the batter.

- 3 tablespoons chia seeds
- ½ cup plus 1 tablespoon water
- 3 cups white whole-wheat, spelt, or (gluten-free) oat flour
- 1 teaspoon baking soda
- 1 teaspoon baking powder
- 1 teaspoon salt
- 1 teaspoon ground cinnamon
- ¼ cup coconut oil, gently melted
- 1 cup coconut palm sugar or evaporated cane juice
- ½ cup flaxseed meal
- 1 tablespoon vanilla extract
- ¾ cup Hemp Milk (page 21) or other nondairy milk
- 2 medium zucchini, grated

1. Preheat oven to 350°F.

2. Lightly oil loaf pans or muffin pans (or line muffin pan with papers).

3. In a large bowl, combine chia and water (to form gel). Set aside.

4. In a medium bowl, combine flour, baking soda, baking powder, salt, and cinnamon with a whisk.

5. In the large bowl, combine the chia gel with sugar, coconut oil, coconut palm sugar, or evaporated cane juice, flaxseed meal, vanilla, and nondairy milk.

6. Slowly mix dry ingredients into wet ingredients. Stir to combine.

7. Mix zucchini into the batter.

8. Divide the mixture among the pans.

9. For loaves, bake 1 hour; for muffins bake 25 to 30 minutes. Bread is done when a toothpick inserted into the center of the loaf or a muffin comes out clean.

10. Remove pans from the oven and turn out onto a cooling rack.

CRUNCHY TOPPED APPLE COFFEE CAKE

MAKES 8 TO 10 SERVINGS

Toasted pepitas and hemp seeds give this delicious brunch treat a protein-rich—and nut-free—crunch.

1 tablespoon chia seeds

¼ cup water

¼ cup shelled pumpkin seeds (pepitas)

¼ cup hemp seeds

¼ cup plus 2 tablespoons coconut palm sugar, divided

¾ teaspoon salt, divided

½ cup olive oil

¼ cup maple syrup

½ cup Hemp Milk (page 21) or other nondairy milk

2 cups white whole-wheat, spelt, or (gluten-free) oat flour

½ teaspoon baking soda

½ teaspoon baking powder

½ teaspoon ground cinnamon

¼ teaspoon ground nutmeg

2 medium apples, peeled and cut into ½-inch dice (approximately 1½ cups)

1. Preheat oven to 350°F.

2. Lightly oil an 8-inch-square baking pan.

3. Combine chia seeds and water in a small bowl (to form a gel). Set aside.

4. Lightly toast pepitas in a dry skillet for approximately 1 minute, or until lightly golden.

5. Using a food processor, pulse together pepitas, hemp seeds, 2 tablespoons coconut palm sugar, and ¼ teaspoon salt.

6. In a large bowl, mix together olive oil, remaining sugar, and maple syrup.

7. Mix in the chia seed mixture and nondairy milk.

8. In a separate bowl, combine flour, ½ teaspoon salt, baking soda, baking powder, cinnamon, and nutmeg using a whisk.

9. Mix dry ingredients into wet ingredients, half at a time, until well incorporated.

10. Mix in apples.

11. Pour batter into prepared pan. Smooth top with a damp spatula.

12. Spread pepita mixture over top.

13. Bake for 30 minutes, or until a toothpick inserted into the center comes out clean.

STRAWBERRY CHOCOLATE CHUNK MINI MUFFINS

*MAKES 24 MINI MUFFINS
OR 12 STANDARD MUFFINS*

You can make these muffins even when strawberries are not in season by chopping frozen strawberries in a food processor or letting them thaw before chopping them by hand.

2 cups white whole-wheat, spelt, or (gluten-free) oat flour

1½ teaspoons baking powder, divided

½ teaspoon salt

½ cup applesauce

½ cup flaxseed meal

¼ cup coconut oil, melted, or canola oil

¾ cup coconut palm sugar or evaporated cane juice

½ teaspoon vanilla extract

¼ cup Hemp Milk (page 21) or nondairy milk

2 cups chopped strawberries

½ cup chocolate chunks or chocolate chips

1. Preheat oven to 350°F.

2. Lightly oil a mini muffin (or standard muffin) pan or line with muffin papers.

3. In a medium bowl, combine flour, 1 teaspoon baking powder, and salt with a whisk.

4. In a large bowl, combine applesauce with ½ teaspoon baking powder.

5. Add flaxseed meal, oil, sugar, vanilla, and nondairy milk to the applesauce. Stir well to combine.

6. Add strawberries to wet ingredients and mix well.

7. Slowly mix dry ingredients into wet ingredients, being careful not to overmix.

8. Mix in chocolate chunks or chips.

9. Spoon batter into prepared muffin pans.

10. Bake approximately 25 to 30 minutes, or until a toothpick inserted in the middle of a muffin comes out clean. (If your muffin pan makes very small muffins—more than 24— reduce baking time accordingly.)

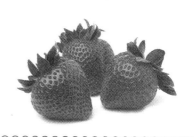

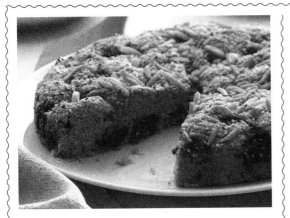

BLUEBERRY COFFEE CAKE

MAKES 8 SERVINGS

Inspired by a traditional Italian almond corn-meal coffee cake, this version, with fresh (or frozen) blueberries, is elevated to "super coffee cake" with the addition of hemp seeds and hemp milk. This cake is truly delicious.

> 1 cup white whole-wheat flour, spelt flour, or (gluten-free) oat flour
>
> 1 cup cornmeal, plus extra for dusting the pan
>
> ½ teaspoon salt
>
> 1½ teaspoons ground cinnamon, divided
>
> 2 teaspoons baking powder
>
> ¾ cup plus two teaspoons granulated sweetener (coconut palm sugar or evaporated cane juice), divided
>
> 1 cup Hemp Milk (page 21) (or other nondairy milk)
>
> ¼ cup applesauce
>
> 1 teaspoon vanilla extract

> 1 teaspoon almond extract (or omit for a nut-free cake)
>
> 1 cup blueberries (fresh or frozen)
>
> 1 tablespoon plus 1 teaspoon slivered almonds (or shelled pumpkin seeds, pepitas, for a nut-free cake)
>
> 1 tablespoon plus 1 teaspoon hulled hemp seeds

1. Preheat oven to 375°F.

2. Grease a 9-inch-round cake pan with coconut oil and dust with cornmeal. Set aside.

3. In a medium bowl, whisk together flour, cornmeal, salt, 1 teaspoon cinnamon, baking powder, and ¾ cup sweetener.

4. In a large bowl, combine hemp milk, applesauce, vanilla, and almond extract, if using.

5. Slowly mix dry ingredients into wet ingredients. Stir to combine.

6. Add blueberries.

7. Pour batter into prepared cake pan.

8. In a small bowl, combine almonds or pepitas, hemp seeds, 2 teaspoons sweetener, and ½ teaspoon cinnamon.

9. Sprinkle nut-and-seed mixture over the top of the cake batter.

10. Bake 25 to 30 minutes, or until a tooth-pick inserted in the center of the cake comes out clean.

11. Let cake cool on a cooling rack for 10 minutes, then turn out onto a plate and flip right side up. Serve warm.

LEMON AMARANTH MUFFINS

MAKES 12

Rosemary pairs with lemon and olive oil to give these muffins a sophisticated taste, while the addition of cooked amaranth provides a tender crumb (it also helps reduce the overall fat—another bonus).

- ¼ *cup olive oil*
- 1 *sprig fresh rosemary or 1 teaspoon dried rosemary*
- 1 *cup white whole-wheat, spelt, or (gluten-free) oat flour*
- ½ *teaspoon salt*
- 1½ *teaspoons baking powder, divided*
- ½ *cup applesauce*
- 1 *cup Basic Amaranth (page 18)*
- 2 *tablespoons fresh lemon juice*
- 1 *teaspoon lemon rind*
- ¾ *cup granulated sweetener (evaporated cane juice or coconut palm sugar)*

1. Preheat oven to 350°F.

2. Lightly oil a standard muffin pan or line with paper liners.

3. In a small saucepan over medium heat, warm olive oil with rosemary for 2 to 3 minutes, or until fragrant. Discard the rosemary and set aside the oil to cool.

4. In a medium bowl, whisk together flour, salt, and 1 teaspoon baking powder.

5. In a large bowl, combine applesauce with ½ teaspoon baking powder.

6. Add olive oil, amaranth, lemon juice, lemon rind, and sweetener to applesauce mixture. Stir to combine.

7. Slowly mix dry ingredients into wet ingredients.

8. Divide batter evenly among muffin cups.

9. Bake for 25 to 30 minutes, or until a toothpick inserted in the center of a muffin comes out clean.

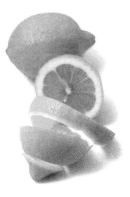

PICK YOUR BERRY MUFFINS

MAKES 12

These muffins are a fantastic vehicle for any berry that's in season, but they're just as delicious as an out-of-season treat, if you use frozen fruit. Either option works beautifully in this recipe.

½ cup amaranth flour

1½ cups white whole-wheat, spelt, or (gluten-free) oat flour

1½ teaspoons baking powder, divided

½ teaspoon salt

½ cup applesauce

½ cup flaxseed meal

½ teaspoon vanilla extract

1 tablespoon apple cider vinegar

1 cup maple syrup

¼ cup coconut oil (gently melted)

1½ cups berries (blueberries, raspberries, strawberry slices, blackberries, or a mix)

1. Preheat oven to 350°F.

2. Lightly oil a standard muffin pan or line with muffin papers.

3. In a medium bowl, whisk together flours, 1 teaspoon baking powder, and salt.

4. In a large bowl, combine applesauce with ½ teaspoon baking powder.

5. Add flaxseed meal, vanilla, vinegar, maple syrup, and coconut oil to the applesauce mixture. Stir to combine. Add dry mixture and stir again to combine.

6. Gently fold berries into batter.

7. Divide batter evenly among muffin cups.

8. Bake for 24 to 30 minutes, or until a toothpick inserted into the center of a muffin comes out clean.

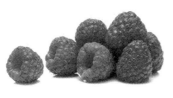

CRUNCHY TOPPED PEAR MUFFINS

MAKES 12

If you don't have any pears on hand, you can substitute apples in this muffin recipe. You'll see why it's a family favorite.

- *2 cups white whole-wheat, spelt, or (gluten-free) oat flour*
- *1 teaspoon baking powder*
- *½ teaspoon salt*
- *1½ teaspoons cinnamon, divided*
- *½ cup applesauce*
- *1 tablespoon apple cider vinegar*
- *½ cup flaxseed meal*
- *¼ cup neutral-tasting oil (canola, grapeseed, or sunflower)*
- *¾ cup granulated sweetener (evaporated cane juice or coconut palm sugar)*
- *¼ cup Hemp Milk (page 21) or other nondairy milk*
- *2 Bartlett or Anjou pears, diced (approximately 1½ cups)*
- *¼ cup hulled hemp seeds*
- *½ cup rolled oats*

1. Preheat oven to 350°F.

2. Lightly oil a standard muffin pan or line with muffin papers.

3. In a medium bowl, whisk together flour, baking powder, salt, and 1 teaspoon cinnamon.

4. In a large bowl, combine applesauce, vinegar, flaxseed meal, oil, sweetener, and hemp milk. Stir to thoroughly combine.

5. Slowly mix dry ingredients into wet.

6. Stir in diced pears.

7. Evenly divide batter among muffin cups.

8. In a small bowl, combine hemp seeds, oats, and ½ teaspoon cinnamon.

9. Evenly top each muffin with seed mixture.

10. Bake 25 to 30 minutes, or until a toothpick inserted in the center of a muffin comes out clean.

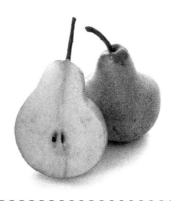

BLUEBERRY SCONES

MAKES 8

These scones are really delicious when served with Blackberry Chia Jam (page 106)

1½ cups white whole-wheat or spelt flour

¼ cup flaxseed meal

2 teaspoons baking powder

½ teaspoon salt

2 tablespoons coconut palm sugar or evaporated cane juice

2 tablespoons cold coconut oil

⅔ cup coconut milk (full fat or light)

½ cup blueberries

1. Preheat oven to 450.

2. In a medium bowl, whisk together flour, flaxseed, baking powder, salt, and sugar.

3. Blend in coconut oil with a pastry cutter or two forks.

4. Stir in coconut milk until just blended in.

5. Stir in blueberries.

6. Shape dough into a flattened disk, approximately six inches across.

7. Place on parchment covered baking sheet.

8. Cut disk into 8 wedges and separate them on the pan.

9. Bake 12 to 14 minutes until puffed and golden.

GLUTEN-FREE SCONES

Recipes for gluten-free scones usually call for oat flour, but in my opinion the moisture in this flour just doesn't yield the right texture for scones. If you'd like to convert the scones in this book to gluten-free, I suggest using an all-purpose gluten-free flour that contains some starch (potato, tapioca, etc.) and add 1 teaspoon xanthan gum to the dry ingredients. Although it is not a whole-grain alternative, this substitution will nevertheless yield scones that have just the right texture and flavor.

PUMPKIN SCONES
TWO WAYS

MAKES 8

At our house, you can never have enough chocolate. These pumpkin scones are delicious when they're studded with chocolate chips or drizzled with a simple glaze. You can also serve them alongside a bowl of soup, without any sweet-flavored additions. There are so many ways to enjoy them!

½ cup amaranth flour

1½ cups white whole-wheat or spelt flour

1 tablespoon baking powder

¾ teaspoon cinnamon

½ teaspoon allspice

3 tablespoons coconut palm sugar (or evaporated cane juice, but the coconut palm sugar really adds depth here)

½ teaspoon salt

¼ cup firm coconut oil (see note)

1 cup pumpkin puree (not pumpkin pie filling)

Optional: ½ cup chocolate chips

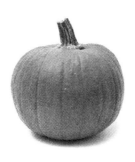

1. Preheat oven to 425°F.

2. In a large bowl, combine flours, baking powder, cinnamon, allspice, sugar, and salt with a whisk.

3. Mix oil into dry ingredients using a pastry cutter or two knives.

4. Thoroughly mix pumpkin into dry ingredients. Mix in chocolate chips if using. (It is easiest to use your hands.)

5. Shape the dough into a disk and cut into 8 triangles.

6. Place triangles on parchment covered baking sheet.

7. Bake for 12 to 15 minutes, or until golden brown and firm to the touch.

GLAZE

2 tablespoons coconut palm sugar or evaporated cane juice

1 teaspoon nondairy milk

1. Thoroughly mix all ingredients.

2. Drizzle on cooled scones.

NOTE: If it's warm in your kitchen and your coconut oil has melted, pop ¼ cup of it in the refrigerator until it firms up.

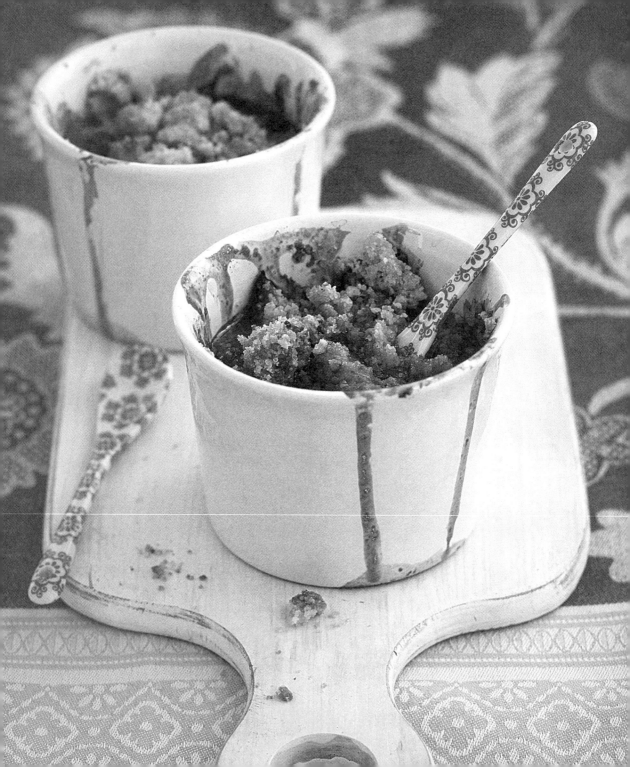

CHAPTER 7

DESETS

Sweet treats can be "super," too, whether you're making a plate of brownies for a bake sale, a fruit crisp for a holiday meal, or a frosty treat on a hot day. When you incorporate powerful ingredients like super seeds into the treats you love, you can nourish the body as well as satisfy the soul. And, since super seeds are loaded with good fiber, they can help fill you up so you don't overindulge at treat time, while the protein, vitamins, and minerals they supply actually add to your overall daily nutrition, rather than loading on empty calories, like so many traditional desserts do. Just because you are powering up your desserts, it doesn't mean you have to sacrifice flavor, as you'll soon discover, once you start rustling up some of the yummy offerings in this chapter. Enjoy!

OPPOSITE: **Strawberry Rhubarb Crisp, page 86**

STRAWBERRY RHUBARB CRISP

MAKES 6 SERVINGS

In the springtime, farmers' markets are loaded with beautiful, pinkish green stalks of rhubarb. The tartness of this hardy plant marries beautifully with the sun-kissed sweetness of late spring strawberries. This recipe calls for apple juice as a sweetener, which helps bring down the amount of sugar that is used in traditional rhubarb desserts.

- *1 cup apple juice*
- *1 tablespoon chia seeds*
- *1 cup rhubarb, thinly sliced (⅛ to ¼ inches thick)*
- *2 cups quartered strawberries*
- *¼ cup coconut oil*
- *½ cup coconut palm sugar or evaporated cane juice*
- *⅛ teaspoon salt*
- *1 teaspoon vanilla extract*
- *½ cup quinoa flakes*
- *¼ cup hemp seeds*

1. Preheat oven to 425°F.

2. Combine apple juice and chia seeds, and let sit for 10 minutes.

3. In a small saucepan, combine apple juice mixture, rhubarb, and strawberries. Bring to a boil.

4. Reduce heat and simmer 10 to 15 minutes, or until rhubarb is soft.

5. In a medium bowl, combine remaining ingredients to make batter.

6. Pour fruit mixture into an 8-inch-square baking pan.

7. Dollop the batter on top of the fruit, using the back of a spoon or damp hands to spread it evenly over the surface.

8. Bake for 40 minutes, or until top is set and lightly browned. Serve with a scoop of vanilla nondairy ice cream.

COCONUT OIL COULD SAVE YOUR SKIN

Coconut oil is not only a superb ingredient for cooking, it is an excellent natural moisturizer. Just rub a little on a patch of rough skin and watch what happens. Some research also indicates that coconut oil may have antimicrobial properties that can help protect skin from infection. Keep coconut oil in a cool place to keep it from liquefying.

* * *

THE BENEFITS OF USING COCONUT OIL

Coconut oil is a great nondairy butter replacement—perfect for baking because it can be substituted 1-for-1 in most recipes that call for butter or oil. Its light coconut flavor enriches all kinds of sweet treats, and it behaves similarly to butter and margarine: At cooler temperatures it is a solid, and in warmer temperatures, it melts into a fat-rich liquid. Also, coconut oil is a whole food, unlike commercial margarine, which is one of the most chemically processed and altered foods on the market. Coconut oil is rich in medium-chain fatty acids, which, research is beginning to indicate, might play a role in lowering blood cholesterol.

SUNFLOWER SEED–HEMP BUTTER SCONES

8 SCONES

If you don't want chocolate in your scone at breakfast, you can substitute raisins or dried cherries for the chocolate chips.

- 1½ cups white whole-wheat or spelt flour
- ¼ cup flaxseed meal
- 2 teaspoons baking powder
- ½ teaspoon salt
- 2 tablespoons coconut palm sugar or evaporated cane juice
- 2 tablespoons sunflower seed–hemp butter (see page 20)
- ⅔ cups non-dairy milk
- 6 tablespoons chocolate chips

1. Preheat oven to 450.

2. In a medium bowl, combine flour, flaxseed, baking powder, salt, and sugar with a whisk.

3. Mix sunflower seed–hemp butter into the flour.

4. Add non-dairy milk, and mix thoroughly.

5. Mix in chocolate chips.

6. Form dough into a disk, approximately 6 inches across.

7. Place on a parchment-covered baking sheet.

8. Cut into 8 wedges and separate them on the pan.

9. Bake 12 to 14 minutes or until puffed and golden.

GOING GREEN WITH SUNFLOWER SEED BUTTER

Sunflower seed butter is a phenomenal substitute for peanut butter or almond butter, if you need your food to be nut- or peanut-free. You can find it in many grocery and health food stores, or you can buy it online. You can also make your own. All you have to do is spread raw, shelled sunflower seeds on a baking sheet and lightly toast them in a 350°F degree oven. After 10 minutes, or until they are thoroughly toasted. With a food processor or high-speed blender, process the warm sunflower seeds until smooth. Add a dash of salt and a drizzle of neutral-tasting oil (canola, grapeseed, or sunflower) until the mixture is smooth.

Here's a wacky detail about baking with sunflower seed butter: It turns green in baked goods when combined with baking soda (or any other alkaline substance). Your cake or cookies will taste delicious, but they'll be teal-colored!

CHOCOLATE CHIP NUT BUTTER SNACK CAKE

MAKES 18 SERVINGS

I am a huge fan of what I call a "snack cake." This is a cake that doesn't need to be frosted or decorated, and you don't need a special occasion to make it. Just cut it up into chunks and eat it with your fingers! These no-frills cakes make any day feel a little fancy. This one is a favorite at our house.

- 2 tablespoons flaxseed meal
- ¼ cup water
- 2 cups white whole-wheat, spelt, or (gluten-free) oat flour
- ½ teaspoon salt
- 1 teaspoon baking soda
- 1 cup Basic Amaranth (page 18)
- 1 cup maple syrup
- ½ cup almond butter or other nut or seed butter
- 1 cup chocolate chips

1. Preheat oven to 375°F.

2. Lightly oil a 9 × 13-inch baking pan.

3. In a large bowl, whisk together flaxseed meal and water. Set aside.

4. In a medium bowl, whisk together flour, salt, and baking soda.

5. To the flaxseed mixture, add the amaranth, maple syrup, and nut butter and stir to thoroughly combine.

6. Mix dry ingredients into wet ingredients, half at a time.

7. Stir in chocolate chips.

8. Spread batter into prepared pan. It will be sticky, so use a damp spatula or your damp hands to spread the batter.

9. Bake 25 minutes, or until a toothpick inserted into the middle of the cake comes out clean.

STRAWBERRY NECTARINE COBBLER

MAKES 9 SERVINGS

If you're craving a taste of summer in the wintertime, use thawed frozen strawberries in this recipe. Can't find nectarines? No problem! You can substitute peach slices for the nectarines. To keep the mix from getting too watery, thaw the frozen fruit and drain off any excess liquid. This cobbler is delicious all on its own or with a scoop of ice cream, sorbet, or nondairy yogurt.

- *¾ cup white whole-wheat flour, spelt, or (gluten-free) oat flour*
- *¼ cup flaxseed meal*
- *½ teaspoon baking powder*
- *¼ teaspoon baking soda*
- *¼ teaspoon salt*
- *¼ cup plus 2 teaspoons coconut palm sugar or evaporated cane juice, divided*
- *¼ cup applesauce*
- *3 tablespoons coconut oil*
- *2 cups nectarine slices*
- *2 cups strawberry slices*

1. Preheat oven to 375°F.

2. In a medium bowl, combine flour, flaxseed meal, baking powder, baking soda, salt, and ¼ cup sugar with a whisk.

3. Mix the applesauce and coconut oil into the flour mixture.

4. In an 8-inch-square baking pan, toss the fruit with 2 teaspoons sugar.

5. Pour batter on top of fruit.

6. Bake 25 to 30 minutes, or until batter is set and fruit is bubbly.

CHOCOLATE CHIP ICE CREAM

MAKES 6 SERVINGS

Chia's natural thickening properties lend creaminess to this ice cream. If you don't have an ice cream maker, you can pour the mixture into ice-pop molds and enjoy a creamy frozen popsicle.

- *2 tablespoons chia seeds, ground*
- *2 15-ounce cans coconut milk (either light or regular)*
- *½ cup maple syrup*
- *1 vanilla bean*
- *1 cup chocolate chips*

1. In a medium bowl, combine chia seeds, coconut milk, and maple syrup.

2. Using a sharp knife, cut the vanilla bean lengthwise. Scrape the center of the bean with a knife or spoon and add it to the mixture.

3. Stir, cover, and chill for at least 1 hour.

4. Freeze ice cream according to ice cream maker's directions.

5. Add chocolate chips in the last couple minutes of mixing the ice cream.

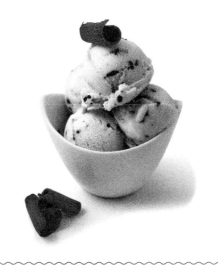

DEVILISHLY GOOD CHOCOLATE CAKE

MAKES 9 SERVINGS

Using parchment paper is the key to getting this moist cake from pan to plate. Otherwise, the chocolate chips that sink to the bottom of the batter will stick to the pan. You can enjoy the cake warm or at room temperature. For an extra treat, serve it with a scoop of Chocolate Chip Ice Cream (page 91) or drizzle some Strawberry Chia Syrup (follow Blueberry Chia Syrup on page 26 and substitute strawberries) over the cake when it's warm. Delicious.

1 cup whole-grain spelt flour

½ cup flaxseed meal

½ cup cocoa powder

1 teaspoon baking soda

½ teaspoon salt

1 cup maple syrup

½ cup olive oil

1 cup brewed coffee (decaffeinated is fine)

2 teaspoons vanilla extract

2 tablespoons apple cider vinegar

½ cup chocolate chips

1. Preheat oven to 375°F.

2. Line the bottom of an 8-inch-square baking pan with parchment paper. Lightly oil the parchment and sides of the pan.

3. In a large bowl, combine flour, flaxseed meal, cocoa powder, baking soda, and salt with a whisk.

4. In a small bowl, combine syrup, olive oil, coffee, and vanilla.

5. Pour liquid ingredients into dry ingredients, and stir to thoroughly combine.

6. Add vinegar, and stir to distribute.

7. Stir in chocolate chips.

8. Spread batter in prepared pan.

9. Bake for 35 minutes, or until center is set.

10. Remove pan from oven and cool for 10 minutes in the pan.

11. Turn cake onto a cooling rack.

CHOCOLATE CHIP COOKIES

MAKES 4 DOZEN

The whole-grain flour and flaxseed meal in these chocolate chip cookies makes them cholesterol-free, and a good source of iron.

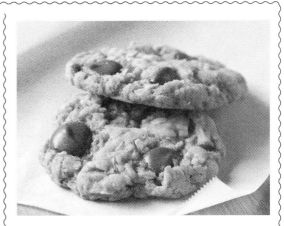

- 2½ cups white whole-wheat, spelt, or (gluten-free) oat flour
- ½ cup flaxseed meal
- 1 teaspoon salt
- 1 teaspoon baking soda
- ½ cup applesauce
- ½ teaspoon baking powder
- ¾ cup neutral-tasting oil (canola, grapeseed, or sunflower)
- 1½ cups coconut palm sugar or evaporated cane juice
- 1 tablespoon vanilla extract
- 1¼ cups chocolate chips

1. Preheat oven to 375°F.

2. In a medium bowl, combine flour, flaxseed meal, salt, and baking soda using a whisk.

3. In a large bowl, combine applesauce with baking powder.

4. Add oil, sugar, and vanilla to applesauce mixture. Mix well.

5. Stir dry ingredients into wet ingredients.

6. Add chocolate chips and stir to combine.

7. Line baking sheets with parchment paper.

8. Drop batter by rounded tablespoon onto ungreased baking sheets.

9. Bake 10 to 12 minutes, or until set.

10. Let cookies cool on baking sheets for a few minutes before removing to cooling racks.

COCOA COOKIE BATTER POWER BITES

MAKES 30

These power bites are perfect for a post-workout pick-me-up. Because they are smaller than a prepackaged nutrition bar, you can eat as many of them as you like. Form the balls all at once, and then store them in a sealed container in the refrigerator for a day or two. You can cut the recipe in half if you don't need so many.

   1 cup pitted Medjool dates

   ½ cup water

   ¼ cup cocoa powder

   1 tablespoon coconut oil

   ¼ cup nondairy milk

   ½ teaspoon vanilla extract

   ¼ teaspoon salt

   ¼ cup nut butter (sunflower seed butter, sunflower seed hemp butter, almond butter, peanut butter, etc.)

  1½ cups quinoa flakes

1. In a food processor or blender, puree dates and water together.

2. In a small saucepan, combine date paste and cocoa powder. Heat while stirring for 2 to 3 minutes.

3. In a large bowl, combine date mixture with coconut oil, nondairy milk, vanilla, salt, and nut butter.

4. Mix in quinoa flakes to thoroughly combine.

5. Cover and chill mixture for at least one hour.

6. Roll mixture into 1-inch balls.

7. Refrigerate until ready to eat.

NATURE'S CANDY

Wonderfully sweet dates are a prominent feature of Middle Eastern cuisine. This isn't too surprising, given that dates, the fruit of the date palm, grow in desert conditions. In the United States, most dates are grown in parts of Arizona and California, where conditions are ideal for their cultivation. Although there are many varieties of dates grown worldwide, only two varieties, Deglet Noor and Medjool, are readily available in the United States. For making date paste, Medjool dates work especially well, since their flesh is plumper than other varieties.

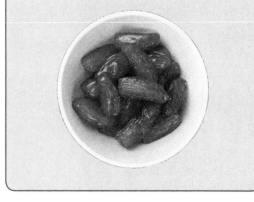

HEMP CHOCOLATE CHIP COOKIE BATTER POWER BITES

MAKES 30

The texture of these power bites is as soft as cookie batter. I like to use mini chocolate chips in this recipe to really spread around the chocolate love.

1 cup pitted Medjool dates
½ cup water
¼ cup hemp seeds
1 tablespoon coconut oil
¼ cup nondairy milk
½ teaspoon vanilla extract
¼ teaspoon salt
¼ cup nut butter (sunflower seed, almond, or peanut)
1½ cups quinoa flakes
½ cup chocolate chips

1. In a food processor or blender, puree dates with water.
2. In a large bowl, combine date paste, hemp seeds, coconut oil, nondairy milk, vanilla, salt, and nut butter.
3. Mix in quinoa flakes thoroughly.
4. Mix in chocolate chips.
5. Cover and chill mixture for at least 1 hour.
6. Roll mixture into 1-inch balls.
7. Refrigerate until ready to eat.

CHOCOLATE BROWNIES

MAKES 9 SERVINGS

A mere two tablespoons of chia in this recipe acts as a fiber-rich, cholesterol-free egg substitute, while a couple of tablespoons of coffee do double duty to bring out a rich chocolate flavor. If you don't have any brewed coffee around, don't worry, you can always use water—the brownies will be very tasty. They're my go-to treat when I need to bring a little something special to a friend's house.

6 tablespoons water

2 tablespoons ground chia seeds

¾ cup coconut palm sugar or evaporated cane juice

¼ cup plus 2 tablespoons neutral-tasting oil (canola, grapeseed, or sunflower)

2 tablespoons brewed coffee

1 12-ounce bag of chocolate chips

1½ teaspoons vanilla extract

1 cup white whole-wheat, spelt, or (gluten-free) oat flour

¼ cup flaxseed meal

½ teaspoon baking soda

½ teaspoon salt

1. Preheat oven to 375°F.

2. In a small bowl, combine water and chia seeds. Let the mixture sit for 15 minutes. Stir to thoroughly mix.

3. In a small saucepan, combine sugar, oil, and coffee. Cook over medium heat until hot but not boiling.

4. Stir half the chocolate chips and the vanilla into the sugar mixture. Stir until the chips are melted. Set aside.

5. In a separate bowl, combine the flour, flaxseed meal, baking soda, and salt.

6. Scrape the chocolate mixture into a large bowl.

7. Stir the chia seed mixture into the chocolate mixture.

8. Slowly mix dry ingredients into wet ingredients. Combine thoroughly.

9. Mix remaining chocolate chips into the batter.

10. Line an 8-inch-square baking pan with parchment paper, long enough to hang over the sides.

11. Pour batter into the parchment paper–lined baking pan. Bake for 30 minutes, or until center is set.

12. Remove pan from the oven and cool in the pan on a cooling rack. Cut into squares when completely cool. Serve with fresh fruit for a lovely dessert.

GRANOLA COOKIES

MAKES 36

These cookies pack all the goodness of super seed–loaded granola into a crunchy cookie that tastes great, travels well, and will quickly become your go-to lunch box and picnic cookie. Enjoy them with a tall glass of iced tea on a hot day or a warm cup of cocoa whenever you feel a chill setting in.

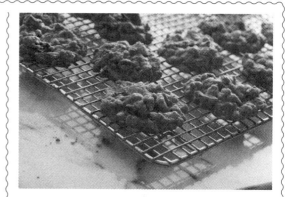

- *1 cup (gluten-free) oat flour, white whole-wheat flour, or spelt flour*
- *½ teaspoon baking soda*
- *½ teaspoon salt*
- *2 cups Fruit-Sweetened Granola (page 30) or Coconut Quinoa Granola (page 34)*
- *¼ cup applesauce*
- *¼ teaspoon baking powder*
- *½ cup coconut palm sugar or evaporated cane juice*
- *¼ cup coconut oil, melted*
- *½ cup chocolate chips or dried fruit*

1. Preheat oven to 350°F.
2. Line cookie sheets with parchment paper.
3. In a medium bowl, whisk together flour, baking soda, and salt.
4. Mix in granola. Set aside.
5. In a large bowl, combine applesauce and baking powder.
6. Mix in sugar and coconut oil.
7. Stir granola mixture into wet ingredients, half at a time.
8. Mix in chocolate chips or dried fruit.
9. Drop tablespoon-size dollops of batter onto cookie sheets.
10. Bake 10 to 12 minutes, or until golden brown.
11. Let the cookies firm up for a minute or two before moving them to a cooling rack to cool completely.

CHOCOLATE ICE POPS

MAKES 4

Avocado is the secret ingredient that makes these ice pops extra-creamy, and it also gives them a punch of healthy fat, fiber, magnesium, and vitamin C. Yum. These luscious ice pops are healthy and delicious at the same time.

1½ cups Hemp Milk (page 21)

⅛ teaspoon salt

½ ripe avocado (Use the other half right away or squeeze with lemon juice to prevent it from browning.)

3 tablespoons cocoa powder

2 tablespoons maple syrup

2 tablespoons brewed coffee (decaffeinated is fine)

1. Blend all ingredients.
2. Pour the mixture into ice-pop molds (see note).
3. Freeze until solid.

NOTE: You can pick up BPA-free ice-pop molds almost anywhere. They come in adorable shapes and colors, and they're not expensive. Best of all, they give you what you need to have a yummy frozen treat that's both sweet and also loaded with fruits and veggies—not to mention super seeds! BPA stands for bisphenol A, an industrial chemical that is found in polycarbonate plastics. Research has shown that BPA can seep into food or beverages from containers that are made with BPA, a concern, since exposure to BPA has been linked, in some studies, to serious health conditions.

SUNSHINE ICE POPS

MAKES 4 SERVINGS

Chia seeds thicken the mixture in these ice pops, making them creamier and a little less icy than the usual frozen treat.

½ cup orange juice, either fresh or from concentrate

½ cup coconut milk

1 cup mango chunks, fresh or frozen

2 teaspoons chia seeds

1. Blend all ingredients thoroughly.
2. Let mixture sit for 15 minutes, then pour into ice-pop molds.
3. Freeze until solid.

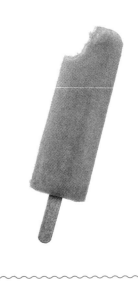

MAKE-IT-YOURSELF
FRESH PUMPKIN PUREE

MAKES APPROXIMATELY 2 CUPS

When the autumn rolls around, my family and I eat a lot of pumpkin goodies. We go through a lot of pumpkin puree, and, as convenient as the canned product is, I've found that making my own pumpkin puree raises the flavor factor by more than a few notches! I love to bake a pumpkin on a cool day, and then transform it into a spectacular treat (such as Pumpkin Pancakes on page 29). Here's the recipe I use. It's super simple.

1 medium pie pumpkin (about 2 to 4 pounds), such as Sugar Pumpkin

1. Preheat oven to 400°F.

2. Wash the outside of the pumpkin.

3. Pierce the pumpkin with a sharp knife in several places.

4. Bake for 45 to 60 minutes. The pumpkin is done when a sharp knife can easily pierce the exterior.

5. When it is cool enough to handle, cut the pumpkin in half.

6. Scoop out and discard the seeds (pepitas) or save them to roast for a snack later.

7. Scoop the flesh into a bowl.

8. Mash with a potato masher.

9. If you're not using the puree right away, store it in a tightly sealed container in the refrigerator for up to three days, or in the freezer for up to 3 months.

PEAR-PUMPKIN CRISP

MAKES 9 SERVINGS

I sometimes serve this crisp as a special breakfast. Thanks to pumpkin, pears, and quinoa flakes, this recipe is packed with iron, fiber, vitamins A and C, and protein—all of which makes me feel a lot less guilty about letting my family indulge a little! And did I mention how delicious it is? For an extra treat, serve this crisp with a dollop of vanilla-flavored coconut-milk yogurt.

> 1 cup pureed pumpkin (canned pumpkin is fine, but not canned pumpkin pie filling) such as Make-It-Yourself Fresh Pumpkin Puree (page 99)
>
> ½ teaspoon ground cinnamon
>
> ¼ teaspoon allspice
>
> 6 pears, such as Bartlett, peeled and thinly sliced (approximately 6 cups)
>
> 1½ cups quinoa flakes
>
> ¾ teaspoon salt
>
> ¾ cup maple syrup

1. Preheat oven to 400°F.

2. Lightly oil a large 9 × 13-inch baking pan.

3. In a large bowl, combine pumpkin with cinnamon and allspice.

4. Add pear slices and toss to cover with pumpkin mixture, then spread in baking pan.

5. In a small bowl, combine quinoa flakes with salt.

6. Add maple syrup and stir to combine.

7. Spread on top of fruit mixture.

8. Bake 35 minutes, or until the crisp is lightly golden on top.

NOT EVERY SEED IS A SUPER SEED

A little healthy skepticism about some seeds is not a bad thing. Apple seeds and apricot kernels, for example, contain small amounts of cyanide. Although you would have to eat a lot of apple seeds to get poisoned, it can be dangerous for children to eat apricot kernels. As a general policy, stick with the super seeds you know.

INDIVIDUAL PUMPKIN PIE PUDDINGS

MAKES 4 SERVINGS

This pudding is wonderfully creamy and smooth—the ultimate comfort food. For the topping, you can use the recipe for granola, below, or either of the recipes on page 30 or page 34.

PUDDING

- ½ *cup coconut milk*
- 2 *tablespoons chia seeds*
- 1 *15-ounce can pumpkin puree or 1¾ cups Make-It-Yourself Fresh Pumpkin Puree (page 99)*
- 1 *teaspoon ground cinnamon*
- ½ *teaspoon allspice*

GRANOLA

- ½ *cup shelled hemp seeds*
- 1½ *cups gluten-free oats*
- 1 *teaspoon ground cinnamon*
- 1 *tablespoon plus 1 teaspoon canola oil*
- 1 *teaspoon vanilla extract*
- ¼ *cup maple syrup*

TO MAKE THE PUDDING

1. In a medium bowl, thoroughly combine all pudding ingredients.

2. Chill in refrigerator for at least 8 hours.

3. To serve, scoop pudding into individual serving dishes and top with granola.

TO MAKE THE GRANOLA

1. Preheat oven to 350°F.

2. Line a baking sheet with parchment paper or a Silpat mat (see note).

3. In a large bowl, combine all granola ingredients.

4. Spread granola on baking sheet. Bake 15 to 20 minutes, or until golden brown, and let cool.

5. Serve with pudding or store in an airtight container and enjoy within 1 week.

NOTE: Silpat is a brand of nonstick baking mat that never needs to be greased and can be used instead of parchment paper.

APPLE CRISP

MAKES 6 SERVINGS

Although apple crisps are delicious served hot with melty vanilla ice cream for dessert, one of our favorite ways to enjoy them is with a generous drizzle of vanilla nondairy yogurt—especially if we're having it for breakfast.

APPLE MIXTURE
    6 *medium-size apples, such as Granny Smith or Pink Lady, peeled, cored, and sliced*
    ¾ *cup coconut palm sugar*
    1 *teaspoon vanilla extract*

TOPPING
    ½ *cup gluten-free oat flour*
    ¼ *cup hemp seeds*
    ¼ *cup rolled gluten-free oats*
    2 *tablespoons neutral-tasting oil (canola, grapeseed, or sunflower)*

1. Preheat oven to 400°F.
2. In a large bowl, combine apple slices with sugar and vanilla. Stir to mix well.
3. In a small bowl combine flour, hemp seeds, oats, and oil into a crumbly mixture for the topping.
4. Spread apple mixture into the bottom of a 1½- to 2-quart baking dish.
5. Crumble topping over apples.
6. Bake 40 minutes, or until the top is crispy and the juices are bubbly.

CHOCOLATE SUNFLOWER SEED BUTTER CHIA PUDDING

MAKES 4 SERVINGS

Cool, smooth chia puddings require no cooking, making them the perfect dessert choice for hot summer days. If you want an even smoother pudding, try using ground chia seeds.

    1 *16-ounce container vanilla-flavored coconut-milk yogurt*
    2 *tablespoons sunflower seed butter*
    2 *tablespoons cocoa powder*
    2 *tablespoons chia seeds*

1. Blend all ingredients together.
2. Spoon mixture into glasses.
3. Refrigerate for at least 1 hour and serve.

CRISPY RICE AND SEED CHOCOLATES

MAKES 12 LARGE CANDIES OR 24 SMALL CANDIES

Homemade chocolates are easy to make and can be customized for any occasion. Festive muffin or candy papers can be used in any standard or mini-muffin pan to make these delicious super-seed chocolates. Wrapped in a cellophane bag and tied with a colorful ribbon, they make a special gift.

> 1 cup chocolate chips
> ¼ cup popped amaranth (see page 19)
> ¼ cup sunflower seeds
> ½ cup crisp brown rice cereal

1. Line a standard muffin pan or mini muffin pan with muffin papers.

2. Heat chocolate chips over medium-low flame, stirring constantly until almost completely melted. Remove from heat and continue stirring until chocolate is completely melted.

3. Stir popped amaranth, sunflower seeds, and rice cereal into melted chocolate.

4. Use a tablespoon to fill a large muffin papers or a teaspoon to fill small muffin papers. Smooth mixture to fill paper cups evenly.

5. Refrigerate candies for at least 1½ hours.

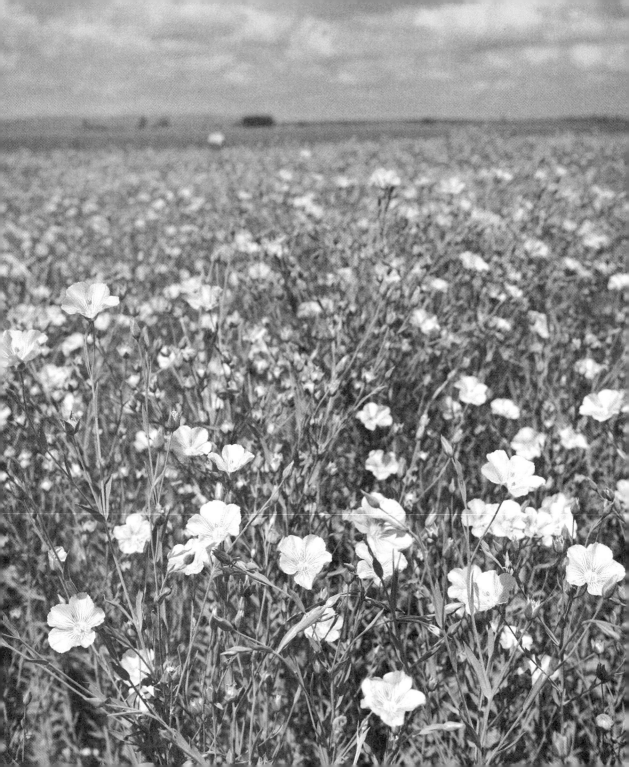

SUPER SEED EXTRAS

Fresh produce and whole grain breads are a tasty first step toward healthy eating. Now you can take these foods to new heights by introducing them to super seed-rich spreads and dips that include powerhouse ingredients such as beans, hemp seeds, and sunflower seed butter. Try adding hemp to both savory and sweet spreads, and enjoy the rich depth of flavor it gives to just about anything you make. You can also mix chia into your favorite veggie dips for a boost of energy, extra fiber, and protein. And if you want to add a luscious dimension to fresh or frozen fruit, you can transform it into a delectable jam in just one hour, by mixing in a little chia. Try the recipe for Blackberry Chia Jam on page 106, and become a convert!

OPPOSITE: **Field of flax in bloom**

BLACKBERRY CHIA JAM

MAKES APPROXIMATELY 1 CUP

> 1 cup blackberries, fresh or thawed
>
> 2 tablespoons apple juice
>
> 1–2 teaspoons maple syrup
>
> 2 tablespoons chia seed

1. Blend well, but keep some texture.
2. Refrigerate for at least 1 hour.

STRAWBERRY CHIA JAM

MAKES APPROXIMATELY 1 CUP

If you want to keep some fruity texture in this chia jam, don't over-blend the strawberries.

> 1 cup strawberries
>
> 2 tablespoons applesauce
>
> 2 tablespoons chia seeds

1. Blend all ingredients together.
2. Refrigerate for at least 1½ hours.

CREAMY DREAMY FRUIT DIP

MAKES APPROXIMATELY 1½ CUPS

If you would like a smoother texture, grind the chia seeds before blending them with the rest of the ingredients. This dip will stay fresh in the refrigerator for 3 or 4 days if you keep it covered. I like serving it with strawberries, bananas, and pineapple.

> 1 container vanilla-flavored
>   non-dairy yogurt
>
> 2 tablespoons orange juice
>
> 2 teaspoons orange zest
>
> ½ teaspoon vanilla
>
> 1 tablespoon chia seeds

1. Mix all ingredients together.
2. Cover and chill for at least one hour.

ITALIAN BEAN DIP

MAKES 1½ CUPS

This Italian take on hummus makes for a delicious sandwich spread as well as a tasty dip for fresh veggies.

  1¾ cups cooked Great Northern Beans
      (or 1 15-oz can, drained and rinsed)
  ¼ cup basil leaves
  2 tablespoons lemon juice
  1 tablespoon olive oil
  2 tablespoons hemp seeds
  1 –2 garlic cloves
    ½ teaspoon salt
    Fresh ground pepper to taste

1. Blend all ingredients together in a food processor or blender.

CREAMY VEGGIE DIP

MAKES ½ CUP

This zippy dip is delicious with cauliflower florets and snap peas.

  ¼ cup Sunflower Seed–Hemp Butter
      (page 20)
  ½ cup plain- or vanilla-flavored
      non-dairy yogurt
    Sriracha to taste (optional)

1. Combine all ingredients.
2. Serve with fresh, crispy vegetables.

METRIC EQUIVALENTS LIQUID

This chart can also be used for small amounts of
dry ingredients, such as salt and baking powder.

U.S. quantity	Metric equivalent
¼ teaspoon	1 ml
½ teaspoon	2.5 ml
¾ teaspoon	4 ml
1 teaspoon	5 ml
1¼ teaspoons	6 ml
1½ teaspoons	7.5 ml
1¾ teaspoons	8.5 ml
2 teaspoons	10 ml
1 tablespoon	15 ml
2 tablespoons	30 ml
⅛ cup	30 ml
¼ cup *(2 fluid ounces)*	60 ml
⅓ cup	80 ml
½ cup *(4 fluid ounces)*	120 ml
⅔ cup	160 ml
¾ cup *(6 fluid ounces)*	180 ml
1 cup *(8 fluid ounces)*	240 ml
1½ cups *(12 fluid ounces)*	350 ml
3 cups	700 ml
4 cups *(1 quart)*	950 ml *(.95 liter)*

METRIC EQUIVALENTS DRY

Ingredient	1 cup	¾ cup	⅔ cup	½ cup	⅓ cup	¼ cup	2 tbsp
All-purpose gluten-free flour	160g	120g	106g	80g	53g	40g	20g
Granulated sugar	200g	150g	130g	100g	65g	50g	25g
Confectioners' sugar	100g	75g	70g	50g	35g	25g	13g
Brown sugar, firmly packed	180g	135g	120g	90g	60g	45g	23g
Cornmeal	160g	120g	100g	80g	50g	40g	20g
Cornstarch	120g	90g	80g	60g	40g	30g	15g
Shortening	190g	140g	125g	95g	65g	48g	24g
Chopped fruits and vegetables	150g	110g	100g	75g	50g	40g	20g
Chopped seeds	150g	110g	100g	75g	50g	40g	20g
Ground seeds	120g	90g	80g	60g	40g	30g	15g

FREQUENTLY ASKED QUESTIONS

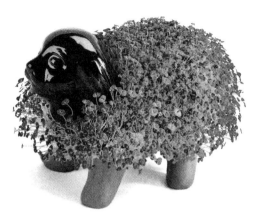

Are the chia seeds you eat the same as the chia seeds from a Chia Pet?

Yes they are! Chia Pets were a popular gift item in the 1980s. They used sprouted chia seeds as the "hair" on a variety of sculptural shapes.

Is there a nutritional difference between white and black chia?

No, they are essentially the same. White chia will blend better in light-colored foods and black chia will be better hidden in dark foods, but you can use whichever chia is most readily available to you.

How can I use flaxseed or chia as an egg replacer?

You can replace one egg in a recipe with either 1 tablespoon flaxseed meal or 1 tablespoon chia seeds mixed with 3 tablespoons water. Let the mixture sit for 10 minutes, and then stir it well before using it.

How can I use flaxseed to replace oil?

You can replace up to half of the oil in recipes for baked goods with two times the amount of flaxseed meal. For example, if a recipe calls for 1 cup of oil, you can reduce the oil to ½ cup and add 1 cup of flaxseed meal. This will give a fiber, protein, and mineral boost to your baked goods.

What's making my baked goods—the ones that include hemp sunflower seed butter—turn green?

Sunflower seeds react with alkaline ingredients (such as baking soda) to turn cakes, cookies, and muffins green. This is purely a cosmetic issue, though, because the results will taste delicious and are good for you.

What is royal quinoa?

Royal quinoa or Quinoa Real, which is grown in the high mountains of the Andes, is a designation of quinoa grown in a specific part of Bolivia, and like the champagne that is produced and bottled in the Champagne region of France, it indicates that this quinoa is the highest quality, and therefore worth a higher price.

Can I grow amaranth in my garden?

Yes. It can grow more than 4 feet high and the foliage is vibrantly colored. The seeds can be harvested in the fall.

Can I eat the leaves of the amaranth plant?

Yes. In the spring, you can add the tender leaves of the amaranth plant to salads. The larger leaves can be sautéed, like spinach or kale, in the summer and fall.

Is the protein in super seeds a good source of protein?

Yes. Protein is made up of amino acids, which are frequently called the building blocks of protein. All of the super seeds included in this book contain a wide range of amino acids, including the nine most important ones for our nutritional needs.

Where is quinoa grown?

Although efforts have been made to cultivate quinoa in North America, Bolivia and Peru still provide the bulk of the world's demand for this popular crop.

Are super seeds gluten-free?

Chia, hemp, amaranth, quinoa, and flaxseed are all gluten-free.

If I have diabetes, should I include super seeds in my diet?

The high fiber content of super seeds slows down digestion and the absorption of carbohydrates, which makes them a useful tool for managing blood sugar.

Is hemp the same as marijuana?

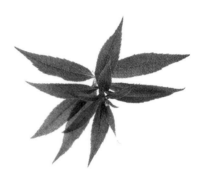

Although hemp and marijuana come from related plants, hemp plants contain negligible amounts of THC, the psychoactive compound in marijuana. Eating hemp seeds, or food that contains hemp, will not make you high.

Can super seeds be part of a weight-management plan?

Due to their high protein and fiber content, super seeds can play an effective role in weight management. They fill you up, slow down digestion (making you feel full longer), and provide you with energy to accomplish your fitness goals.

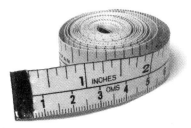

Where should I store super seeds?

Storing super seeds in a cool environment will help them stay fresh. Flaxseed and hemp seeds are particularly sensitive to heat, and should be kept in the refrigerator or freezer to prevent them from going rancid. Although quinoa and amaranth can be kept in a sealed container in the pantry, storing them in the refrigerator will extend their life.

Can I freeze prepared quinoa or amaranth?

Yes, you can prepare more quinoa or amaranth than you need for a particular recipe and freeze it in small portions. You can then thaw it for use in another recipe, as a side dish, or even for breakfast.

Why does flaxseed need to be ground?

Flaxseed has a hard coating that protects the inner seed. The nutrition in the kernel can't be accessed until the shell is cracked. Grinding the seeds into meal makes the inner nutrients accessible.

How can I grind my own flaxseed meal?

A nut-and-seed grinder is a great way to grind your own flaxseed meal from whole flaxseed. If you don't have one, a clean coffee grinder is a practical alternative.

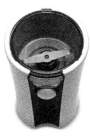

Does chia need to be ground first, in order for the nutrients to be absorbed?

No. Unlike flax, chia does not have a hard external coating. Its nutrients are equally accessible whether chia is used whole or ground.

Can I make my own quinoa or amaranth flour?

You can grind your own quinoa and amaranth into flour by using a high-speed blender, or in small batches by using a nut-and-seed grinder. Store flour that you're not using in a sealed container in the refrigerator for up to 1 week or in the freezer for up to 3 months.

RESOURCES

There are so many wonderful resources online for healthy cooking. Here are some of my favorites:

Kim's Welcoming Kitchen

www.welcomingkitchen.com

Whole foods–based recipes that are allergen-free, gluten-free, and vegan.

Cooking Quinoa

www.cookingquinoa.net

Website includes hundreds of quinoa-based recipes.

Dreena's Plant-Powered Kitchen

www.plantpoweredkitchen.com

Whole-foods, family-friendly recipes.

Spabettie

www.spabettie.com

Beautifully photographed whole-foods, vegan, and gluten-free recipes.

Ricki Heller

www.rickiheller.com

Gluten-free, vegan, and sugar-free recipes featuring whole foods.

Healthy Blender Recipes

www.healthyblenderrecipes.com

Easy-to-prepare whole foods using blenders, food processors, and mixers.

Recipe Renovator

www.reciperenevator.com

Traditional favorites made healthier.

Azchia

www.azchia.com

Website packed with chia information, recipes, research, and ordering opportunities.

Go Dairy Free

www.godairyfree.com

Website focusing on living dairy-free, and featuring recipes, nutrition information, and tips.

NUTRITION INFORMATION RESOURCES

Do you want to know more about the food you're eating? These resources will help you understand the nutrient breakdown of the foods you love and introduce you to some new, healthy options as well.

SELF Nutrition Data

http://nutritiondata.self.com

Nutrient information for foods and ingredients hosted by SELF magazine.

The World's Healthiest Foods

www.whfoods.com

Recipes and nutrient information for healthy eating.

Office of Dietary Supplements, National Institutes of Health

http://ods.od.nih.gov

Nutrient research presented for lay people.

The Whole Grains Council

www.wholegrainscouncil.org

Though not technically grains, quinoa and amaranth are included as part of the Whole Grains Council website.

HELPFUL EQUIPMENT RESOURCES

Cuisinart

www.cuisinart.com

Full line of kitchen appliances, including nut-and-seed grinders, blenders, food processors, immersion blenders, ice cream makers, and more.

KitchenAid

www.kitchenaid.com

Full line of kitchen appliances, including stand mixers, blenders, coffee grinders, waffle makers, food processors, and more.

Black and Decker

www.blackanddeckerappliances.com

Full line of kitchen appliances, including blenders, food processors, coffee grinders, waffle makers, and more.

These are some of my favorite cookbooks that use super seeds creatively.

Welcoming Kitchen: 200 Delicious Allergen and Gluten-free Vegan Recipes, Kim Lutz (Sterling, 2011)
I use flaxseed and quinoa in many of the recipes in Welcoming Kitchen. This book has 200 recipes that are safe for almost everyone, because they are free of the top eight allergens, and are gluten-free and vegan, as well.

Chia: The Complete Guide to the Ultimate Super-food, Wayne Coates, PhD (Sterling, 2012)
This book highlights chia's role in fitness and weight loss, as well as providing facts, trivia, and recipes using chia.

The Quintessential Quinoa Cookbook, Wendy Polisi (Skyhorse, 2012)
The recipes in this book, by the creator of the Cooking Quinoa website, use quinoa for every occasion.

Superfood Kitchen, Julie Morris (Sterling Epicure, 2012)
This beautiful book features super seeds, along with a host of other super foods.

Let Them Eat Vegan, Dreena Burton (DaCapo, 2012)
The plant-based recipes in Let Them Eat Vegan highlight whole foods and whole grains, including various super seeds.

The Blender Girl, Tess Masters (Ten Speed, 2014)
These quick-and-easy vegan recipes come together with the help of a blender, food processor, or mixer.

Quinoa, amaranth, hemp, flaxseed, and chia are available in many large grocery stores and natural food markets. There are also many natural food suppliers online. These are some of the more popular companies that sell super seeds.

Bob's Red Mill
www.bobsredmill.com
A full line of super seeds and super-seed flours.

Nutiva
www.nutiva.com
Hemp, chia, and coconut products.

Navitas Naturals
www.navitasnaturals.com
Chia, hemp, flaxseed, and a host of other super foods.

Ancient Harvest
www.quinoa.net
Quinoa, quinoa flour, quinoa flakes, quinoa pasta.

Manitoba Harvest
www.manitobaharvest.com
Hemp seed

Arrowhead Mills
arrowheadmills.com
Quinoa, amaranth, and flaxseed.

Spectrum
spectrumorganics.com
Chia, flaxseed, and flax and hemp seed blend.

Living Harvest
livingharvest.com
Tempt line of hemp foods, including hemp milk and hemp tofu.

Pacific Naturals
pacificnaturals.com
Hemp milks.

RECIPES BY SUPER SEED

INDEX

NOTES

NOTES

NOTES

NOTES

Kim Lutz is a Chicago-based author and founder of Kim's Welcoming Kitchen (welcomingkitchen.com), a Top 25 Food Allergy Mom Blog and Top 25 Vegetarian/Vegan Mom Blog. She is a contributor to the influential website VegNews.com and co-author of *The Everything Organic Cooking for Baby and Toddler Book* and *The Everything Guide to Cooking for Children with Autism*. Lutz has been featured in the *Chicago Sun-Times*, *Chicago Parent*, and on WGN-TV, among other media. *Welcoming Kitchen: 200 Delicious Allergen and Gluten-free Vegan Recipes*, published by Sterling in 2011, received a Silver Nautilus Award in 2012, and has received glowing reviews from *Library Journal*, *VegNews*, *Living Without*, and *Vegetarian Journal*.

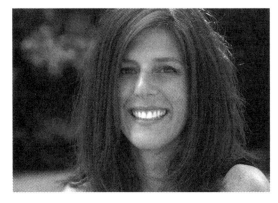

Photo by Sandra Wettig

ACKNOWLEDGMENTS

If it takes a village to raise a child, it takes a community to help bring a cookbook into being. Friends and family tasted, tested, and critiqued these recipes. My family lived with a disaster in the kitchen, not to mention a distracted mom!

I am most grateful to Jennifer Williams, my editor, who has believed in me and shown me enormous patience and caring. I would not have this book without her guidance and support.

These recipes are better because of the time and effort put in by the best team of recipe testers ever: Ilene Mash, Julie Han, Karen Plumley, Valerie Hedge, and Julie Goding. I also had some enthusiastic tasters: Steve, Casey, and Evan Lutz (of course); the Sagami clan, Laura, Rob, Matthew, Isabel, and Samantha; Ilene and Jeff Mash; Dana Kissinger; the Bermingham-Snyder ladies, Stacy, Katie, Izzy, and Maddy; Gavin and Noah Han, and anyone on the playground I could pin down!

Thank you for the professional expertise of two dedicated dietitians, Megan Hart and Lara Field.

The only reason I can even think about writing a book is because of the love and support that I get from my family.

CREDITS

Courtesy of Chia Pet ®, registered trademark of Joseph Enterprises, Inc: 110

Getty images: Maximilian Stock Ltd., 51; Ian O'Leary, 25

Istock Photo: Abbie Images, 80; Monika Adamczyk, 31; Alex5248, 5; Alina555, 26; Aluxum, 98; Akhilesh, 94; AmbientIdeas, 55; Ansonsaw, 46; Ralph Baleno, 14; Bluestocking, 77; Cjrfoto, 16; Creativeye99, 83; Philip Dyer, 112 (left); Elenathewise, 104; Erickson Photography, 60; Tina Fields, ix; Floortje , 10; Sarsmis, 84; Sitan Magnus Hatling, 3; Jamesmcq24, 39; Jsemeniuk, 111; Julichka, 28; Ka-ching, 4; kcline, 72; Lujing, 38; Maurusone , 7;

Night And Day Images, 93; Ntstudio, 79; Ockra, 42; David Orr, 6; PixelBay, 91; Princess Dlaf, 20; softservegirl, 97; Subjug, 24; Syolacan, 54; Alasdair Thomson, 62; Valentinarr, 87; John Woodcock, x; YinYang, 41

Bill Milne: 2, 22, 27, 36, 43, 48, 52, 64, 68, 70, 78

Shutterstock: Chay, 81; Mr. Hanson, 17, 112 (right); Anna Kucherova, 47; Ellen Mol, 56

Stock Food: Gräfe & Unzer Verlag / Michael Brauner, 8

ALSO AVAILABLE IN THE SUPERFOOD SERIES!

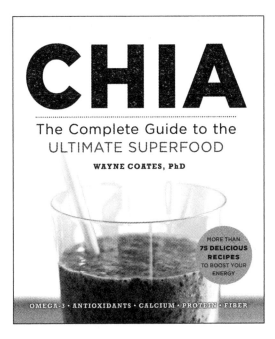

CHIA

The Complete Guide to the Ultimate Superfood
Wayne Coates, PhD, with Stephanie Pedersen
978-1-4027-9943-3
$14.95 ($17.95 Canada), in paper with flaps

Chia is the little miracle seed for anyone trying to lose weight, stay healthy, and enhance well-being. Used by the Aztecs for centuries, it's a gluten-free natural appetite suppressant that helps regenerate muscle, sustain energy, and balance blood sugar. This definitive work explains all you need to know about chia, and provides a comprehensive daily strategy for weight loss with delicious recipes!

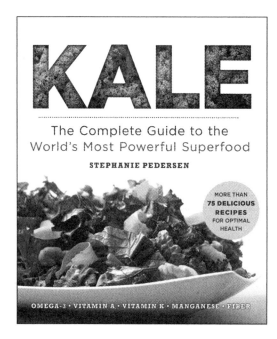

KALE

The Complete Guide to the World's Most Powerful Superfood
Stephanie Pedersen
978-1-4549-0625-4
$14.95 ($15.95 Canada), in paper

From farmers and foodies to celebrity chefs—everyone's gone mad for kale! For those eager to get in on this healthy, tasty trend, here is a fun-to-read, one-stop resource for all things kale, including more than 75 delicious recipes to entice, satisfy, and boost well-being. Stephanie Pedersen, a holistic health counselor, provides dozens of tips for making kale delicious and desirable to even the most finicky eater.